Beauty
from Afar

Beauty
from Afar

**A MEDICAL TOURIST'S GUIDE TO
AFFORDABLE AND QUALITY COSMETIC CARE
OUTSIDE THE U.S.**

Jeff Schult

STC HEALTHY LIVING

Stewart, Tabori & Chang
New York

NOTICE: This book is intended as a reference guide, not as a medical guide or manual for self-treatment. The information is intended to help you make informed decisions about your health. The recommendations in this book should only be used with the consent and consultation of your primary care physician. If you are under the care of a physician for any medical condition, do not use any information in this book without first discussing it with your doctor.

Editor: Debora Yost
Design: 3+Co.
Production Manager: Kim Tyner

Published in 2006 by
Stewart, Tabori & Chang
An imprint of Harry N. Abrams, Inc.

Library of Congress Cataloging-in-Publication Data
Schult, Jeff.
Beauty from afar: the medical tourist's guide to affordable and quality
cosmetic surgery outside the United States/Jeff Schult.
p. cm.
Includes bibliographical references and index.
ISBN 1-58479-486-0
1. Surgery, Plastic—Economic aspects.
2. Medical care, Cost of.
3. Medical tourism.
4. Surgery, Plastic—Economic aspects—United States.
5. Medical care, Cost of—United States. I. Title.

RD119.S348 2006
617.9'5—dc22
2006000032

Cover photograph: Andre Cezar/Getty Images

The text of this book was composed in Din and Helvetica Neue.

Printed in the United States of America

10 9 8 7 6 5 4 3 2 1

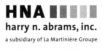

HNA
harry n. abrams, inc.
a subsidiary of La Martinière Groupe

115 West 18th Street
New York, NY 10011
www.hnabooks.com

DEDICATION
For Kellen Michael Schult,
the best son a dad could have
—then, now, and always.

CONTENTS

FOREWORD

At first blush, it may seem a bit odd that a board-certified plastic surgeon living and practicing in the United States is writing a foreword for a book detailing the ins and outs of getting cosmetic treatments outside of this country. What's next? Major airlines offering insight into bus travel? At the risk of being called a heretic, however, there are several reasons why I think education about cosmetic medicine abroad is useful and why this book, *Beauty from Afar*, can be helpful for people considering surgery outside the United States.

First, let me say that I support the cautious position of the American Society of Plastic Surgeons (ASPS), detailed in this book, on travel abroad for cosmetic surgery. It is sound advice that I feel is inarguable. At the same time, the ASPS has been very good about including and cultivating the input and instruction of very talented surgeons from around the world. Their techniques are frequently included in ASPS journals and educational meetings.

On a personal note, I have been extremely fortunate to have spent time training with very gifted physicians practicing outside the United States, among them Dr. Ivo Pitanguy in Brazil. The techniques that I acquired while observing these doctors are an integral part of my practice today and are used on an almost daily basis. I have personally seen quality surgical skills outside of our borders.

When we talk about travel abroad for medical services, we are almost always involving an aspect of medical economics. We Americans know that we have an extremely competent medical system. But we also know that in relation to the rest of the world, we have the most expensive. Health care in America can come at a very high cost. This means that, at times, many Americans are unable to afford the highest level of health-care services that they feel they may want or deserve. This is true of the aesthetic medical field as well. While my advice would always be to have your surgery done domestically if you can afford it, there are many people who simply would not be able to have a procedure done if they had to pay U.S. prices. In today's global market where multiple companies and individuals are outsourcing to save on costs, it comes as no surprise that this phenomenon has surfaced in the medical industry.

Ultimately, however, quality and safety must be the top priority, whether you are seeking medical attention here or abroad. Unfortunately, in the United States as well as in other countries, there seems to be no shortage of unscrupulous practitioners who portray themselves as experts in their field, but who have never completed a recognized training or credentialing process. The medical experience for a patient is daunting enough, even in a qualified and legitimate familiar environment. Stepping over the border for equally qualified and legitimate care requires guidance. That's why *Beauty from Afar* is so essential. This book provides individuals the necessary tools to make an informed decision when seeking out individual health-care options. Its solid principles apply to anyone searching out quality health care, whether across town, a border, or the ocean…

John J. Corey, M.D.
Aesthetic Surgeon in Private Practice
Scottsdale, Arizona
U.S.A.

AUTHOR'S NOTE

Throughout the research and writing of *Beauty from Afar*, I communicated with and consulted many surgeons, doctors, nurses, and other health-care professionals. I talked to and consulted many more people than those mentioned or quoted in this book, having had to pick and choose each step of the way. Readers should not assume that any particular doctor or medical facility has my endorsement just by fact of their appearance in these pages. That which serves the general narrative of this book should not be taken as more than that. In no way do I mean to suggest, for example, that the surgeons to whose work I refer are better at what they do than many others who are unmentioned. They are offered as illustrative examples and are among those who have the most experience in medical tourism. From their collective individual experiences, from the published news reports about medical tourism of the last decade, from extensive research online, and from collateral reading of what few books touch upon the subject, I was able to assemble a more general picture of what individual prospective medical tourists should seek out, and what they can expect to find.

Similarly, that I mention companies that cater to patients who wish to travel abroad for surgery should in no way be construed as endorsing the quality of their services. Again, they are examples, a few chosen from many fledgling enterprises. It is my personal judgment, based on lengthy experience as a journalist and virtually none with startup companies, that those I selected have a stronger chance than most of succeeding in the long run, but I have no way of knowing for sure.

In the interests of full disclosure, readers should also know I have accepted no remuneration, fee, or discounted services from any business or individual mentioned in this book. I owe meals to a couple of people, perhaps, but owe favorable or preferential treatment to no one and made no bargains regarding treatment in return for interviews or access to facilities. Many of those I did interview were allowed to review draft text of *Beauty from Afar* to check the accuracy of my reporting, and I thank them all for their time and diligence. The end product is solely my responsibility.

Many people have asked me why I chose to write about the specific countries that I did. Fine low-cost medical services and talented, highly qualified surgeons exist in many others. All along, however, I was determined to provide information about countries that are currently the most accessible and inviting to medical tourists, the ones where the U.S. and European markets are targeted and courted. Certainly, one can find excellent plastic surgeons and medical facilities in many countries that are unmentioned in this book. If you prefer going to one of them, don't take my neglect as a sign of my disapproval. Do your homework, choose wisely, and have a great trip.

ACKNOWLEDGMENTS

I'd like to simply ask anyone who'd like to be acknowledged to bop over for dinner some night as soon as I'm settled in again somewhere, assuming that you don't mind eating take-out. We can sit around and talk and I can thank you properly and fulsomely. But it would be a pretty empty gesture unless I left some directions or at least an address, neither of which I can anticipate right now. The only thing I know for sure is that we will do this again some time. That's fair warning for those who found me less than entertaining while writing a book than they would have thought.

I started writing acknowledgments when the book was only half done, which seems pretty presumptuous, but it was about at that point that I realized that there really would be a *Beauty from Afar* and that there would be people to thank for that. First, thanks to everyone who always believed that I would write a book—Mom and Dad, my brothers, assorted friends over the years. That was a lot of damned pressure, you know? No wonder it took me until I was 49! But it's okay, I forgive you enough to thank you lots, for everything, all along the way. In particular, I owe Frances Kuffel for saying that I would be good at this in such a way that I believed her, and for her encouragement, faith, and support as a friend. I have called this faith a curse, on occasion, but thank her for it regardless.

More graciously, perhaps, I'd like to thank Susan Campbell, who gave me the idea that going to Costa Rica for dental work might be a fine magazine story, which it was, and Stephanie Summers, the best managing editor that the *Hartford Courant's Northeast* magazine could hope to have had, for publishing that really long story. Whoever heard of a 10,000-word piece about dental work?

Next, chronologically, I want to thank Beth Bruno for introducing me to my agent, Linda Konner, and Linda for persevering on my behalf through the perhaps inevitable 20 or so rejections, until finding an editor who agreed with us that this book was a good idea. That editor, Debora Yost at Stewart, Tabori & Chang, later told me that there are a lot of books about cosmetic surgery and that they all say the same things (which explains, somewhat, the rejections). But she was the only acquisitions editor who read my proposal and realized that my book was not about cosmetic surgery, but was much more about traveling abroad for medical care, a topic about which she knew almost nothing. She warmed to it, and I am grateful. Many thanks also to Lisa Andruscavage, whose questions and assiduous copy editing both sharpened and smoothed my best early efforts.

I am humbly grateful to all the surgeons, doctors, and medical professionals around the world who contributed to this project by sharing their knowledge and experience, and hope that they find the result did them justice individually and collectively. I have a heightened appreciation, in particular, for the deep, shared commitment to well-being that they hold universally, wherever they may practice, under whatever conditions.

Finally, I'd like to thank the patients, too many to count, who shared with me their experiences in traveling abroad for medical care and cosmetic surgery; and I hope, as I know they do, that the publication of *Beauty from Afar* will illuminate the path along which they traveled and show the way for others to come.

Seeking Beauty from Afar: How I Got My Smile Back

became a "medical tourist" in the early spring of 2004, when I traveled to Costa Rica for major dental work I could not afford in the United States. I use the term medical tourism, with the benefit of hindsight, as a catch phrase for the unusual business of traveling a long way for health care. It did not gain currency in the media until later the same year. At the time, I considered myself...as what? Not a tourist. More of an exile, perhaps. Though there are certainly terrific dentists in the United States, I couldn't afford them. I was on the outside of the health-care system looking in.

My teeth and gums had deteriorated prematurely in my forties to the point where smiling was no longer an instrument of charm. I needed what dentists call full-mouth reconstruction. Insurance companies generally call it unnecessary and would rather wait a few years before contributing to the cost of what by then would be an entirely necessary full set of dentures. In any case, there was not an insurance plan in the world that would cover the $18,000 to $30,000 that a United States dentist would have charged for my full-mouth reconstruction—not unless I'd lost my teeth in a horrible accident, as opposed to simply having them wear away over time. I know. I shopped around.

All this I knew in 2001. By 2004, I had mostly resigned myself to having bad teeth. A quirky grin had become my all-purpose expression of approval. If my misshapen teeth appeared in a photograph, I touched them up with a bit of virtual dentistry. I hoped that what was left of my teeth would last me, functionally, until I was eligible for Medicare. I admit that the molars were still fine for chewing, that the ragged fronts could still tear food. "Let vanity go, you're 48 years old," said a voice in my head. I avoided looking at my teeth even when brushing them and tried not to be bitter.

On the evening of February 16, 2004, I was reading the latest messages on the "Interesting People (IP)" e-mailing list, an influential Internet forum hosted by Professor David Farber, often called, without much exaggeration, the Father of the Internet. The topic was the outsourcing of technology jobs overseas. Jim Warren, a computer professional and long-time online activist, went off on a mild tangent about how it is not just technology jobs that are leaving the country.

"Many Americans fly to Bangkok to get needed—or simply desired—medical and dental procedures...everything from crucial transplants and sex reassignments to cosmetic surgery and liposuction. The surgery, hospital, and drug costs are 'almost nothing' by comparison to U.S. medical, surgical, and hospital charges."

Warren told of a good friend who had a laparoscopic adrenalectomy—an operation to remove a benign tumor of the adrenal gland—that would have cost $30,000 or more in the United States. In Thailand, she paid 100,000 baht—a little less than $2,600. The quality of care, he said, was outstanding.

Immediately, I was thinking about my teeth again. It had never occurred to me to shop outside of the United States for dental care. Thailand! It sounded a little crazy.

Nevertheless, 3 months later, after a lot of reading, correspondence, and consideration, I was reclining in a dental chair not in Thailand but in San José, Costa Rica! The cost of my full-mouth reconstruction fit inside my credit card limit. Six root canals, 14 crowns, and 10 days later, I was heading for home with perfect teeth and a dazzling smile for less than half of what it would have cost me at home.

I chronicled my journey for *Northeast*, the Sunday news magazine of Connecticut's *Hartford Courant*. The article over time provoked more gratitude than anything I had written in 20 years of journalism. It also got a chilly reception from dentists in Connecticut. "Hey, maybe the *Courant* could get a cheaper reporter from Botswana," was one of the more memorable gibes.

"You were very brave," a friend said. She meant, "I wouldn't have done it. You always were a little crazy." But I knew that I wasn't crazy, and I also knew I wasn't alone. While in Costa Rica, I'd met dozens of people who were in the country for health care—mostly cosmetic surgery and dentistry—and learned that San José had, for years, cultivated a reputation as the "Beverly Hills of Central America." It was an open secret, decades old, spread first solely by word of mouth and later via the Internet.

JURASSIC PARK IT'S NOT

I remember what I had known about Costa Rica before I had started thinking of it as a place where I might get fine dental work done inexpensively. Not a lot—but perhaps about as much as did my friend. In fact, I am somewhat embarrassed to admit that I had not been 100 percent sure that Costa Rica was not an island, though I vaguely recalled that Costa Rica was somehow prominent in the 1991 bestseller *Jurassic Park*. I had to look it up. Michael Crichton's ill-fated island was located off the coast of Costa Rica. It is hardly a friendly reference point for a potential visitor. In fact, it seemed to cause a little embarrassment when I mentioned it to a few Costa Ricans, as though they worry that North Americans might actually fear that there are T-Rexes and raptors in the outskirts of San José. But in the book, there is a casual mention of Costa Rica as a destination for those interested in having cosmetic surgery.

> *Bowman, a thirty-six-year-old real estate developer from Dallas, had come to Costa Rica with his wife and daughter for a two-week holiday. The trip had actually been his wife's idea; for weeks Ellen had filled his ear about the wonderful national parks of Costa Rica, and how good it would be for Tina to see them. Then, when they had arrived, it turned out that Ellen had an appointment to see a plastic surgeon in San José. That was the first Mike Bowman had heard about the excellent and inexpensive plastic surgery available in Costa Rica, and all the luxurious private clinics in San José.*

This, in 1991! I asked Michael Crichton, through his publicist, how he had come to include this aside. Though *Jurassic Park* is, of course, fiction, it seemed unlikely that the author would have wholly invented his characterization of Costa Rica. The response I received was that it was a long time ago; Crichton didn't remember how he had come to include the passage. In any case, I felt as though I was more than a dozen years late to a party. I found out later that Costa Rican plastic surgeons have been catering to U.S. patients since at least the late 1970s. Who knew? Lots of people, obviously; and at the same time, hardly anyone.

"We can't say it's a new thing," I told my editor at *Northeast*, Stephanie Summers. "It's been going on for a long time." She was unimpressed. "It's new to our readers," she said.

And it was. Months after the story ran I was still getting e-mail. I put the article online, more or less as a roadmap for others who might want to think about undertaking a similar journey. I thought—there's a book in all this. And there was. Dentistry in Costa Rica barely touched the surface of the cosmetic work being done outside the United States—the same quality, just for a lot less money.

A NOSE JOB IN IRAN?

I first focused on the bigger picture, which was plastic and cosmetic surgery in Costa Rica and elsewhere, and soon found myself swimming in a sea of Internet message boards. Mexico—was it safe? Had anyone been to Malaysia? Did South Africa make any sense at all? Why Spain for weight-loss surgery? Nose jobs in Iran, tummy tucks in Colombia, sexual reassignments in Thailand, new boobs in Brazil…it seemed that in every corner of the globe, plastic surgery was being performed for fees dramatically less than those charged by doctors in the United States and Europe, and it was even being done in places prospective patients could consider going to for a vacation.

Still, it was something one had to know about to find. It was a phenomenon, perhaps even a trend, but small—in fact tiny—when measured against the number of people who *don't* leave the country for cosmetic surgery. It didn't even really have a name yet, though the mainstream media made periodic attempts to label it. "Lipotourism" was tried on for size (notably by *The New York Times*), but it didn't really stick, describing, as it did, mostly a quick trip for fat suctioning and not much else. I'd run across "medical tourism" and used it once in an article, but it wasn't in common usage. "Health tourism" was another borderline misnomer. As time passed, the term "medical tourism," as uncomfortable as it is to some people, caught on.

IT'S SO...FOREIGN

The mainstream media in the United States didn't really know what to do with the story. It was so...*foreign*...and always seemed tainted with desperation and a little craziness. No one seemed to know how many people were getting on airplanes and traveling abroad for inexpensive plastic surgery. Doctors in the United States, when asked, uniformly warned against the practice.

If you paid attention only to newspaper, magazine, and television reports emanating from the United States in 2004 regarding traveling outside the country for cosmetic or plastic surgery, you would reasonably conclude, in fact, that anyone who did so successfully was simply lucky. First-person stories such as my own were few and far between. The bulk of the reporting fell into two broad categories:

1. **Horror stories.** If someone went overseas for plastic or cosmetic surgery and came back dissatisfied, disfigured, or, very occasionally, in a box, it was news. As a journalist, I fully empathize with why this was so. Such cautionary tales of *This could happen to you!* are a staple of journalism everywhere.

2. **Novelty stories.** I would call them success stories, but they were rarely offered as such. As opposed to the this-could-happen-to-you tales, these were stories that portrayed traveling abroad for surgery as though the patient (and the reporter) had stumbled upon something exotic, something cutting edge, not quite ready for prime time. Again, as a journalist, I empathized. As my editor at *Northeast* said, "It's new to our readers."

I was reminded of the last phenomenon on which I'd done significant research and reporting, the rise of the Internet in the mid-1990s. Reading and watching the mainstream media at that time, one could be forgiven for thinking that the new medium was notable only for spreading pornography (horror) and creating instant millionaires (novelty.) Eventually—and it took several years—the media found context, understood what was happening, and started explaining it better.

The same sort of comprehension regarding medical tourism started to evolve in 2004. As I continued the routine of research, reading dozens of e-mails a day, plowing through message-board postings, checking for the latest news, home and abroad, I watched the story change. It would not have happened so fast without the Internet. In fact, it wouldn't have happened at all without the Internet. But change it did, rapidly.

COMPETITION FOR THE UNITED STATES

The new context emerged out of the Far East and spread from government officials and hospitals to business journals. In India, Thailand, Malaysia, and other countries, medical tourism was not a fad; it was a business sector, an important part of the new Asian economy. Sure they were doing inexpensive boob jobs, and if that was all it was, maybe the story wouldn't have changed.

But they were also doing inexpensive open-heart surgery and opening brand-new hospitals that rivaled any in the United States. The story grew in 2004 and spilled out over the Internet. In 2005, it splashed across the front pages and onto cable and network news in the United States. Two premises about traveling abroad for surgery now co-exist, uneasily.

The first is that traveling abroad for surgery or medical care is unacceptably risky and should be avoided. This is certainly the general view of the medical profession in the United States, and it is shared by the bulk of the population. If one subscribes to this premise, the idea of traveling abroad to save money on elective procedures such as plastic or cosmetic surgery sounds especially foolhardy, as in *Who cares if it's cheap? You don't even need it!* or *Why not save up until you can afford to do it right?*

The second premise is that the rest of the world, or at least some of it, has caught up with the United States in quality of medical care and facilities, and that going abroad for lower costs can be the best option, especially for high-cost elective and uninsured procedures and surgeries. Under this view, going abroad for plastic and cosmetic surgery is not a last, desperate resort but a best affordable option for the hundreds of thousands, even millions of people who desire such procedures annually. If the doctors and facilities overseas are up to U.S. standards but the prices are 30 to 80 percent less (even factoring in travel expenses), what is so hard about that decision?

There is truth in both premises, of course; and I considered that I was unprepared to write *Beauty from Afar* until I could argue impressively for either. One thing—perhaps *the* one thing—that supporters of either view would agree on is that consumers of medical services should do their homework and be as informed as humanly possible about their options.

To that end, I offer *Beauty from Afar*, representing, as it does, about 18 months of day-in, day-out homework and research into traveling abroad for medical care, particularly plastic and cosmetic surgery, and dentistry. This book is intended as an introduction to medical tourism and as a guide to those who might want to consider traveling abroad for health care, whether as a best affordable option or as a last resort.

CHAPTER 1

Medical Tourism: Here, There, and Everywhere

t is April 2004, and I am having breakfast with a few new friends at Las Cumbres Inn outside San José, Costa Rica. Sandy, perhaps 45, a Californian, is nearly recovered from her nips and tucks, and is contemplating having her teeth bleached. "Might as well do it while I'm here," she mutters, knowing she'll be heading home in a few days.

Vicki, also fortysomething, and a self-described vagabond, wears dark glasses to cover the swelling from the work done on her still-healing eyes. She is a U.S. citizen who has lived frugally but comfortably in a Costa Rican village for most of the past 11 years. She is thinking she is going to need to get a job again, soon.

Nina looks like she had been in a car wreck. She has had a face-lift, a neck lift, a "medium chemical peel," and perhaps some other "work" that does not fix in my memory. She shows me the estimate she had gotten from a cosmetic surgeon in New York City for the major procedures she wanted. It came to $22,420: $18,000 for the face and neck lift, $2,100 for an operating room fee, $1,320 for post-operative nursing care, and $1,000 for anesthesia.

Her entire bill in Costa Rica will come to $5,700, she says. On this morning, she wonders if she will ever again look anything like she had looked before, let alone better or younger. We assure her that she will, and later, we are proven right.

Me? I tell Sandy about my dentists, Josef Cordero, D.D.S., and Telma Rubinstein, D.D.S., childhood sweethearts who went to college and dental school together, got married, and have spent more than 20 years building an international practice. Sandy decides to go with me in the van that day to see if they can squeeze her in for a teeth bleaching. They can. We all feel pretty smart, in the way people do who have a shared secret.

***

Fast forward to April 2005, a year later. My phone rings at home, a little too early. "Did you see *60 Minutes* last night?" the voice asks. I hadn't, actually; instead, I had been sitting in a gymnasium in West Haven listening to my son play clarinet with his high school concert band. But I had known what *60 Minutes* was doing. Weeks before, Ruben Toral, who is responsible for public relations at Bumrungrad Hospital in Thailand, had told me that CBS had been filming there.

Later, I watch a tape of the show and am frankly astonished that it portrays medical care in Thailand and India as being of the highest quality, and at a fraction of the cost of the same care in the United States. *The lid is off*, I think. It is not a new story to me, of course; but that *60 Minutes* had done it raised the credibility level. If there was something awful about medical tourism, anything especially dangerous about going overseas for health care, surely they would have found it? Millions of people saw the show. Hundreds of thousands of people, at least the ones who have already been overseas for health care—felt vindicated, a little less crazy. The next morning, I read, on a prominent mailing list on the Internet, this comment:

> This could turn out to be one of the most important stories 60 Minutes *has ever produced. First, because it addresses one of the most critical issues in America: rising health-care cost (combined with the uninsured), and second, because the show's audience are the prime consumers of these services: the aging baby-boomers. While I can see that it might take a few years for flying to Asia for major surgery to catch on, I predict that insurance companies will eventually find a way to use these options to force U.S. health-care providers to lower their prices. (Of course, then the battles in Congress will start...)*

Whatever sense I had of being privy to a secret vanished.

***

It is May 2005, Memorial Day weekend. Fabio Zamprogno, M.D., of Vitoria,

Brazil, stands in a hotel conference room in Orlando, Florida, huddled with a few patients and business associates. "How did I do?" he asks. The question has nothing to do with surgery. He wants to know about his presentation to prospective North American patients. Better than last year, he is told, better than in Las Vegas. His English is much improved. Fabio smiles. In the past 2 years, he has done full-body makeovers on more than 100 North Americans who had weight-loss surgery; perhaps no United States surgeon has done so many. Nearly 400 separate operations, in all—at prices one can not find in the United States. Some of the women sport "Body by Fabio" t-shirts. He does not have to ask about his proficiency with a scalpel, with a laser, with a liposuction canula. At this moment, he is more concerned with his marketing skills.

***

It is July 2005. In Pacific Palisades, California, Didi Carr Reuben's schedule is booked for the rest of the year; she is taking reservations for 2006. Didi sets up cosmetic surgery appointments—not for surgeons in nearby Beverly Hills, but for Alejandro Lev, M.D., in Costa Rica. Dr. Lev's credentials are impeccable, and his prices for face-lifts, tummy tucks, breast implants, and the like are typically a fifth of what his peers in ZIP code 90210 might charge. Didi might not be popular in Beverly Hills, but she is adored by the guests at her "Sleepaway Camp for the Terminally Vain," and that is what matters to her.

PATIENTS GOING ABROAD: A BURGEONING INDUSTRY

The story of modern medical tourism is, at one level, also part of the story of the changing global economy—of giant and accelerating shifts in the production of goods and services to nations that have lower costs than the United

The story of modern medical tourism is also part of the story of the changing global economy.

States and Western Europe. The catch-all phrase for this is "globaliza-tion," and it represents, depending on whom one listens to, anything from the end of civilization as we know it to the last, best hope of mankind. The truth, as always, is more complicated, though that is of little solace to workers in the United States whose jobs have been outsourced, whose factories have been off-shored, who are still trying to figure out just exactly how "free trade" is helping them.

For the estimated 42 million people in the United States who lack adequate medical insurance,[1] however, the globalization of quality medical care and services actually is one of the benefits of free trade. And the avail-ability overseas of comparatively inexpensive elective procedures, including plastic and cosmetic surgery, gives Americans willing to travel outside the country options to which they are turning in increasing numbers.

Medical care, however, is not like manufacturing textiles or CDs or writing computer programs or providing technical support via telephone. In the United States, and everywhere else, the first requirement of a medical-care system is that care be available locally, and the second is that it is available swiftly in an emergency. No one is going to go abroad for a simple check-up, for a flu shot, to have a cavity filled, to set a broken bone—not unless they live near a border and it is con-venient to do so. Increasing num-bers of Americans willing to travel overseas for certain kinds of treatments and surgeries will not have a radical impact on the gen-eral delivery of health-care services in the United States anytime soon. In some areas, the effect is ambiguous; medical tourism is a back-up sys-tem, a safety valve for the American health-care system.

> Medical tourism is part of the shift of goods and services to nations that have lower costs than found in the United States.

That an uninsured North Carolina man would have heart valve surgery in a state-of-the-art hospital in India with top-flight surgeons and eight registered nurses tending to his needs for $10,000 instead of in a hospital near his home for $200,000, as reported by CNN in January 2005, does not deprive the hospital in the United States of $200,000 in revenue. The man didn't have insurance and he didn't have the money. Having surgery in India was a way to save or extend his life in a way that he could afford. His only choice in the United States was to wait until he had a heart attack so that he could be treated on an emergency basis. Assuming he survived, sticky financial negotiations that might lead to his bankruptcy would be left until later.

> An uninsured North Carolina man had heart valve surgery in a state-of-the-art hospital in India with top-flight surgeons and eight registered nurses tending to his needs for $10,000 instead of in a hospital near his home for $200,000.

Medical tourism, in the short run, provides a similar safety valve for the public health-care systems of Canada and Western Europe where the problem is not so much cost as it is accessibility. People needing or wanting nonemergency medical treatment can wait months to see a doctor. Canadians may even venture to the United States for care, despite the cost, to avoid average waits that were as high as 17.9 weeks in 2004.[2]

In June 2005, the *Deccan Herald News Service* of India reported that the largest holiday tour operator in Great Britain, Thomas Cook, and the Apollo Group of India were in advanced negotiations over all-inclusive medical tourism packages. Those close to the deal speculated that the number of Britons who might travel to India for health care could rise from 400 or so annually into the tens of thousands, should the trip become sufficiently routine.

U.S. HEALTH CARE AND SPIRALING COSTS

There is no denying that a public rush to embrace medical tourism could have significant impact for the more expensive or overburdened health-care systems of the West, particularly for the United States. The health-care system in the United States has been considered to be in crisis for much of my adult life due to rapidly increasing costs. Health-care spending in the United States reached 15 percent of Gross Domestic Product (GDP) in 2003, even with 42 million or so individuals uninsured.

The United States, by far, has the most expensive health care in the world by almost any measurement. It may have the best quality of medical care in the world, though that is a contentious statement. What is most important right now for the future of medical tourism in the United States is that most Americans believe they have access to the finest doctors, the most advanced medical technology, and the top facilities in the world. They believe this at a gut level; it is something they have been told all their lives. They hold this conviction only slightly less absolute and dear, perhaps, than they do the notion that the United States is the best and/or greatest country in the world.

We Americans, deep down, have difficulty believing that individual doctors, dentists, surgeons, and medical facilities abroad can be every bit as good as the ones at home. It is mostly because we have been instilled with a belief in the superiority of the U.S. medical system, mostly by people who are part of that system. It is close enough to the truth that it is a difficult notion, psychologically, to abandon. It is a part of the American mindset.

> At some level, we are profoundly concerned about the quality and cost of medical care in the United States, which leaves open the door to the possibility of medical tourism.

At some level above that gut feeling, however, we are profoundly concerned about the quality and cost of medical care in the United States, which leaves open the door to the possibility of medical tourism. We may believe we have the best, but we also think it is not nearly good enough, and that it costs way too much.

According to a poll released in November of 2004,[3] 55 percent of Americans were dissatisfied with the quality of health care compared to 44 percent 4 years earlier; just 17 percent said the quality of U.S. care was improving. Another survey, this one released in June 2005,[4] found that 45 percent of Americans were "very worried" about having to pay more for health care and insurance. In fact, more respondents were "very worried" about rising health-care costs than having an income that wasn't keeping up with rising prices (40 percent); not being able to pay rent or the mortgage (24 percent); losing money in the stock market (19 percent); being the victim of a terrorist attack (18 percent); or losing a job (17 percent).

Despite these numbers, I am glad not to have to challenge the notion that U.S. medical care is generally the best in the world. After a year of researching medical care around the world, I have greater esteem for the U.S. medical community than I did previously, and I count myself among the minority that thinks that quality in the United States is generally getting better.

I think we have terrific doctors and surgeons, the finest medical technology, bar none, and more of the finest medical facilities than any other country. You might disagree. But that is really an argument for politicians, doctors, and health-care policy analysts. Whether the quality of health care in the United States is getting better, or worse, or is treading water, is an interesting question, certainly. But does a patient care about the overall quality of the $1.7 trillion American medical system when making a personal decision about what doctor to go to or what surgeon to choose? The answer would seem to be immaterial to someone who is making the personal, one-on-one choice as to what doctor to see or what surgeon should operate.

It would seem to be the case, anyway, unless and until one is considering choosing a doctor or surgeon outside of the United States. For most people, a powerful caution kicks in. It certainly did for me.

DEAR DR. RUBINSTEIN...

When I contemplated traveling abroad for dental work, it took me a month of research on the Internet before I was finally ready to make a direct inquiry. A month—and that was just to feel confident about choosing a country from which I would select a dentist! I chose Costa Rica over Thailand because proximity to the United States played a big role in my thinking. I don't want to go too far if I don't have to. This, from someone who had thought nothing of taking off for Africa for a year, at age 20.

There was a wealth of information available on dentists and dentistry in Costa Rica at the time, more so than anyplace else (except for the United States, of course). I wrote to the aforementioned Telma Rubinstein, D.D.S., of Prisma Dental in San José, Costa Rica, on February 16, 2004. Prisma had a Web site. I confess I chose them as first contact because they had a female dentist. I felt sure I would have a lot of questions, and my instinct was that a woman would be more likely to be patient with me.

Dear Dr. Rubinstein,

I am writing to inquire about having cosmetic dental work done at your practice in Costa Rica.

My dentist here in Connecticut, two years ago, had taken a mold of my bite and recommended, as I recall, eight or 12 porcelain crowns. I must say I concur with his opinion. My teeth are quite worn and small, at 47 years of age. I also have a badly chipped front tooth. I could send you digital photographs, if you'd prefer to see that way.

My dental insurance at the time would not cover any of the considerable fee, however. I now find myself without dental insurance at all, but I recently heard that practices such as yours could do a fine job on the work I require at a significant savings. What can you tell me beyond what I have read on the Internet? How would we proceed?

Thank you for your time,

Jeff Schult

I never had to write to another dentist in Costa Rica or elsewhere. During the next 6 weeks, I peppered Telma, as she asked me to call her, with more than 20 e-mails filled with questions about her credentials and experience, my teeth, prices, travel and accommodations, and Costa Rica in general, and she patiently answered every one.

Still, I didn't really make up my mind until after I asked her if she had any problems with my writing a magazine article about my experience. She had no qualms at all, and I took that as a sign of her complete confidence in her ability. I realized that I already knew more about Telma Rubinstein than I had ever bothered finding out about any doctor or dentist who had treated me in the United States.

Later, I felt kind of bad about having been so difficult. "I put you through the wringer," I told her when we finally met.

She laughed. I had been easy, she said, compared to many of her prospective patients from the United States: "Some of them, Jeff, they ask me so many questions that I feel I have been stripped naked!"

Since then, I have heard similar stories from doctors, dentists, and surgeons around the world who treat patients from the United States. It is not my intention to challenge the notion. As I've already stated, I believe that the United States has the highest quality of medical care in the world, the most and the best medical facilities, the highest level of technology, and the most stringent regulations and standards.

Does that mean that all doctors and dentists and surgeons in the United States are better than all of their peers abroad, or even that most of them are? I do not think even the most xenophobic member of the American Medical Association (AMA) would dare make such an assertion in intelligent company. Even the most vociferous critics of medical tourism acknowledge that there are many fine doctors, surgeons, and dentists around the world working in facilities that are

> Even the most vociferous critics of medical tourism acknowledge that there are excellent doctors and facilities in nations other than the United States.

as modern as anything in the United States. But the official party line of the medical establishment in the United States is: Traveling abroad for surgery is generally far more risky than having surgery in the United States. Bad things are far more likely to happen. You shouldn't do it.

The recent history of medical tourism in the United States suggests that more and more prospective patients for elective surgery, particularly candidates for cosmetic and plastic surgery, are rejecting the medical establishment's No. 1 considered wisdom in this matter. By far, the No. 1 reason they are doing so is cost. Aesthetic and cosmetic surgeries are elective services, paid for out-of-pocket by patients. Wealthy patients are not so price-sensitive, but procedures are no longer for just the well-to-do. The demand for aesthetic and plastic surgery has skyrocketed in the United States and around the world. U.S. surgeons performed three times more face-lifts in 2004 than in 1992; nearly eight times as many people had liposuction.[5] A whole new business in so-called minimally invasive procedures (like Botox and injectible fillers) was born in the space of a few years. In 2004, U.S. cosmetic plastic surgeons performed more than 9.2 million separate procedures. The most visible sign of the broad acceptance of aesthetic and cosmetic surgery in mainstream society was the emergence of several popular (and controversial) reality television shows such as *Dr. 90210*, *The Swan*, and *Extreme Makeover*. *The Swan* and *Extreme Makeover* were short-lived, but that they made it to television at all was a sure sign that plastic surgery is no longer seen as just for the affluent. Americans of more modest means also want to look good— but price matters.

100,000 FELLOW TRAVELERS—OR MORE

Today, with access to the Internet, the millions of prospective and actual cosmetic surgery patients in the United States can be remarkably well-informed before ever setting foot in a surgeon's office. They're familiar with the procedures; they've seen before-and-after pictures. The Internet and television have supplemented traditional word-of-mouth marketing of cosmetic surgery, and many U.S. doctors build their practices substantially through their Web sites.

But the Internet also opened up this vast U.S. market to aesthetic and cosmetic surgeons abroad. And in increasing numbers, they are going after the U.S. market directly.

How many people from the United States are actually going south of the border (or anywhere else) to save money on liposuction, face-lifts, tummy tucks and the like? In recent news stories, the conventional line, almost to the point of cliché, was "no one knows." I have been told by several U.S. surgeons who cared to speculate that the numbers are negligible; however, these have been the same surgeons who are most concerned about (or opposed to) people going overseas for surgery. Some doctors and journalists have guessed it to be in the "low thousands."

This is almost certainly bad guesswork, though it all depends on who and how one wishes to count. Consider, and do the arithmetic along with me:

- **Costa Rica, the "Beverly Hills of Central America,"** where there are perhaps 35 to 40 cosmetic surgeons who work primarily on patients from the United States. The best and most experienced are busy constantly, and some will do several surgeries a day. These board-certified surgeons each handle as many as 40 to 50 U.S. patients a month. Even accounting for slackers, one cannot put the annual total at less than 5,000. It could be double that or more. A prominent surgeon I know puts the total at more than 20,000.

  One can speculate conservatively that a similar number of people visit Costa Rica for just dental work, as I did. There are a lot more dentists, according to one surgeon, and there is some overlap, as many patients will have both plastic surgery and dental work done on the same trip. Many procedures are also done by non-board-certified physicians and surgeons.

- **Brazil, a mecca for cosmetic and plastic surgery with a reputation that precedes and, in much of the world, overshadows that of Beverly Hills.** There are more than a million Brazilian-Americans in the United States. The population has tripled since 1990. Perhaps there was a time when only hundreds or a few thousand U.S. residents traveled to Brazil for cosmetic surgery annually, but that time is past. Brazilian surgeons are polishing their English and their Web sites and building new facilities. Count another 10,000 and growing.

- **Mexico, the most telling of all.** There, more than 900 board-certified plastic and cosmetic surgeons ply their trade. Despite a stream of cautionary and negative news reports about the practice through the years, undoubtedly far more U.S. residents visit Mexico for cosmetic and plastic surgery than any other country. There are more than 30 million Mexican-Americans in the United States, as a receptive base market. Mexican surgeons advertise in the United States and even visit our country regularly on marketing expeditions, mostly in the South and West. It is not reasonable to guess that "a few thousand" U.S. residents head for the border annually for cosmetic surgery. I venture an educated estimate that the number is at least 40,000.

  Tourists seeking liposuction or face-lifts do not declare their intentions at the border, and I have run across only a few doctors and surgeons abroad who can give a good estimate of the number of U.S. patients they see themselves, let alone an aggregate number for their country. But the number for Mexico adds up quickly. I'm told that perhaps half the doctors do little or no work on patients from the United States. Still, if the other half averages two U.S. patients per week, the total would come to nearly 50,000. This does not account for cosmetic dental work or the number of patients who get cosmetic surgery from non-board-certified physicians. It also ignores the fact that there are hundreds of thousands of U.S. citizens living in Mexico, perhaps as many as a million, who presumably are likely to seek medical care, including cosmetic surgery, from local doctors and surgeons.

- **The Dominican Republic**, another medical tourism destination that has been vilified, more often than not, in the popular media in the United States. There are approximately 60 busy cosmetic surgeons in and around the capitol, Santo Domingo. For many of them, more than half of their patients come from abroad, mostly from the United States. Moreover, there are more than a million Dominicans residing in the United States, at least 600,000 of them in the New York City metropolitan area alone.

  Dominican surgeons travel to New York regularly to make

presentations to prospective patients. The prices of even the best, most-qualified surgeons in the Dominican Republic for common surgical procedures are 50 to 70 percent less than what is charged in the United States. Business is booming. It is not unreasonable to guess that board-certified plastic surgeons in the Dominican Republic, plus other doctors and surgeons who perform cosmetic procedures, see at least 10,000 patients a year from the United States, not including dental patients.

- **The rest of the world**. A "few thousand" more from the United States travel to other **Central** and **South American countries**, all of which are represented in the United States by growing immigrant groups. Destinations in the **Far East** are growing in popularity; **Eastern Europe** and **South Africa** are more popular with western Europeans as places to go than they are with Americans, but surgeons in those countries have only just begun competing for the huge North American market. And **Malaysia** and **Thailand** are both increasingly popular destinations. Add another 10,000 to 20,000 to the total, easily.

I am comfortable, then, in conservatively guesstimating the number of U.S. citizens currently traveling abroad for plastic and cosmetic surgery at something in the high five figures, approaching 100,000. This would be about 5 percent of the 1.7 million estimated cosmetic surgeries performed in the United States.

I don't have a similar feel for the total number of U.S. patients who go abroad for dental care, other than to suspect that it is similarly substantial. Certainly, at least a dozen major dental practices in Costa Rica thrive on serving the U.S. market.

An assertion that the number of U.S. residents, mostly women, who would travel abroad for cosmetic surgery might be rapidly approaching 100,000 annually, or

> Until the last decade, the story of what is now called medical tourism was of foreigners going to the United States for sophisticated treatment.

even higher, will no doubt nettle some doctors and surgeons in the United States. Yet how are we to get a grip on the phenomenon (or "problem," if that is your point of view) if we do not attempt to get a handle on its size? Until the last decade, the story of what is now called medical tourism was mostly about people in other countries coming to the United States for sophisticated medical treatment, if they could afford it. And the traffic has by no means completely reversed. Many thousands of people still come to the United States for health care, including cosmetic surgery. Almost certainly, far more money comes into the United States from abroad to pay for medical care than leaves the country.

TIP OF THE ICEBERG—AND A TREND

Global competition for health-care dollars is relatively new. The balance is shifting. From the perspective of many health-care professionals in the United States, Canada, and the nations of Western Europe, this is unsettling. It highlights some of the deficiencies in Western medical systems: in the United States, high costs and a high number of uninsured; and in Canada and Western Europe, long waits and similarly high costs for elective procedures. At one time, only a small number of people from the developed nations went abroad for inexpensive plastic surgery, while a large number of wealthy people from countries with lesser medical care came to the West for advanced care, treatment, and surgery. The estimated 100,000 people (and growing) who now leave the United States annually for plastic surgery only represents the tip of an iceberg for medical tourism as big business.

There are already large success stories that have legitimized this point of view. **Bumrungrad International Hospital in Bangkok, Thailand, is the best known;** in 2004 it boasted treating more than 350,000 patients from 150 countries. **India** is hurrying in the same direction, projecting that medical tourism could be a $2.2 billion business by 2012. Put this way, it sounds huge and economically threatening to the United States and its medical-care system. One can imagine that 10 years from now, the lion's share of the U.S. cosmetic and other elective surgery businesses will be offshore; that U.S. insurers and Health Maintenance Organizations (HMOs) will be putting a hefty percentage of nonemergency-care patients with expensive treatment or surgical needs on airplanes out of the country rather than sending them to local doctors, hospitals, and surgeons. This is a highly exaggerated scenario.

Medical tourism, as such, does not represent a substantial immediate threat to the medical system of the United States, or any other country for that matter. What, after all, is a few billion dollars compared to the $1.7 *trillion* spent on health care in the United States each year? The billions represent a small shift in revenues in a worldwide multi-trillion dollar health-care system. By serving the uninsured and the underinsured in the United States and by providing an alternative to long waits for treatment or surgery in Canada and Western Europe, medical tourism in a sense is augmenting the health-care systems of developed countries, filling and bridging gaps, providing another safety net.

As for aesthetic and cosmetic surgery—the "tip of the iceberg" for the medical tourism phenomenon— overseas surgeons are filling a need. Time and time again, I have heard from surgeons in Mexico, Brazil, Costa Rica, and the Dominican Republic: We are not taking patients away from U.S.

> Medical tourism does not represent a substantial threat to the medical system in the United States.

plastic surgeons. Our patients come to us because they cannot afford U.S. prices. If not for us, they would not have surgery at all.

There are many doctors and surgeons in the United States who would prefer that medical tourism just go away. And cosmetic surgeons, personally and through their membership organizations, have thus far expressed most of the public concern and opposition. This is understandable, but there are degrees of opposition, and one would be mistaken to think that all are of the same mind. It is reasonable to suspect that, as time goes on, more medical professionals in the United States will take a less U.S.-centric position and, generally, accept that they have an international community of peers.

Just a few months after I returned from my dentistry adventure in Costa Rica, I had an appointment with my ophthalmologist. I am extremely nearsighted and have been from an early age. I've worn contact lenses for 36 years, which seems an impossibly long time. In the last several years, my eyes changed such that I was perilously close to requiring bifocals or, as an alternative, reading glasses to wear with my contact lenses. My eye doctor, on this visit, told me that I was an excellent candidate for Lasik eye surgery. I knew what Lasik was, certainly. I knew a lot about it. What lifelong myopic didn't read up on that when it came out? But I had never before been told I was a good candidate for it.

"It's improved a great deal in the last two years," she told me, in response to my questioning about the procedure's reliability and success rate. "They've refined it. We probably won't see it get much better than it is right now, not anytime soon."

I knew that Lasik surgery costs more if one is severely nearsighted. She nodded when I guessed the cost. "Yes, you'd probably be paying around $4,000."

I hesitated, and then told her my Costa Rica story, the short version. And I asked, point blank, if she would help and support me if I chose to get Lasik surgery done overseas. Would she work with the foreign doctor, help me get the best care I could? Because I didn't have $4,000 for Lasik surgery.

She looked me right in the eye.

"Absolutely," she responded, firmly, surprising me a little. And we had a long talk about where would be the best place to go. My ophthalmologist had a slight preference for India, though we agreed, laughing, that as a second-generation Indian, she perhaps has a prejudice.

MEDICAL TOURISM: A MOVING TARGET

Among the great advantages of the Internet as a publishing medium is that it can be updated quickly and efficiently, and among the loveliest examples of this is Wikipedia, the free online encyclopedia. "Medical tourism" was born as an entry in Wikipedia in June 2004[6]; the initial entry read:

Medical tourism is the practice to visit countries with low prices and buy services in their private hospitals.

By September 2005, the entry had expanded to:

Medical tourism is a term that has risen from the rapid growth of an industry where people from all around the world are traveling to other countries to obtain medical, dental, and surgical care while at the same time touring, vacationing, and fully experiencing the attractions of the countries that they are visiting. A combination of many factors has lead to the recent increase in popularity of medical tourism: exorbitant costs of health care in industrialized nations, ease and affordability of international travel, favorable currency exchange rates in the global economy, rapidly improving technology and standards of care in many countries of the world, and most importantly the proven safety of health care in select foreign nations have all led to the rise of medical tourism. More and more people are traveling abroad as an affordable, enjoyable, and safe alternative to having medical, dental, and surgical procedures done in their home countries.

Medical tourists are generally residents of the industrialized nations of the world and primarily come from the United States, Canada, Great Britain, Western Europe, Australia, and the Middle East. But more and more, people from many other countries of the world are seeking out places where they can both enjoy a vacation and obtain medical treatment at a reasonable price.

Currently, medical tourists are traveling in large numbers to India, the East Indies, and South America—three places where the quality of health care is equal to anywhere else in the world and yet the cost is significantly lower. These regions also offer numerous options for touring, sightseeing, shopping, exploring, and even lounging on sun-drenched beaches. Although India, the East Indies, and South America are currently the most popular choices for medical tourists, the industry is growing so rapidly that more and more countries and medical centers around the world are beginning to tailor services aimed specifically at medical tourists, and the expec-

tation is that the options for where medical tourists can choose to travel will continue to increase at a rapid pace.

A myriad of options exist for medical tourists—from purely elective procedures such as rhinoplasty, liposuction, breast augmentation, orthodontics, and Lasik, to more serious and life-saving procedures such as joint replacements, bone marrow transplants, and cardiac bypass surgery. Medical tourists can now obtain essentially any type of medical or surgical procedure abroad in a safe and effective manner for a fraction of the cost that they would face in their home countries.

The cost savings are enormous. For example, for the same price as a week-long vacation for two in Hawaii that includes airfare and boarding and lodging, a couple can travel to the natural and lush beauty of Kerala on India's southeast coast to include airfare, boarding and lodging, personal tour guide/concierge, and Lasik corrective surgery for two.

The average cost of private heart surgery in the United States is $50,000. That same operation with comparable rates of success and complications costs only $10,000 in the finest and most state-of-the-art hospital in Bombay. A bone marrow transplant that costs $250,000 in the U.S. costs only $25,000 in India. Large price disparities such as these exist across the board for numerous medical and surgical procedures. And because of favorable currency exchange rates for medical tourists, the costs associated with accommodations, food, shopping, and sight-seeing are similarly very favorable.

Phenomena come and phenomena go, of course. But the evidence is that medical tourism will be with us for a while. It has just begun.

Notes

1   National Center for Health Statistics, 2004 National Health Interview Survey. Early Release of Selected Estimates.

2   Fraser Institute (Vancouver, B.C.) 14th annual edition of "Waiting Your Turn: Hospital Waiting Lists in Canada" (2004).

3   Harvard School of Public Health Survey conducted with the U.S. Agency for Healthcare Research and Quality in Rockville, Maryland, and the Kaiser Family Foundation, based in Menlo Park, California. Nov. 2004.

4   Kaiser Family Foundation, Kaiser Health Poll Report, June 2005.

5   American Society of Plastic Surgeons Statistics. at www.plasticsurgery.org.

6   http://en.wikipedia.org/wiki/Medical_tourism, Sept. 2005.

CHAPTER 2

Comparing Quality, Comparing Costs

f ever there was a day that America was going to be persuaded that traveling abroad for inexpensive plastic surgery is foolhardy and dangerous, it was July 2, 2004. The story, a result of a news conference called by the city of New York, made the front page of *The New York Times*; it made every major newscast. *A Warning on Cut-Rate Surgery Abroad*, was the *Times*' headline. At least nine women in New York and seven more elsewhere had been diagnosed with serious infections, all traced to their having had cosmetic surgery in the Dominican Republic.

The *Times* attributed the problem to "what has apparently become a phenomenon among New York City's Latinas: cosmetic surgery conducted in the Dominican Republic after being arranged through beauty salons in Washington Heights and other city neighborhoods." The city's health commissioner, Thomas Friedman, M.D., and other officials called the bilingual news conference in the city's Washington Heights section for the express purpose of warning New Yorkers (and anyone else who would listen): Don't even think about going out of the country to have plastic surgery—especially to the Dominican Republic.

"It is so important to get the message that·something that is cheap can be very costly," said New York City Councilman Miguel Martinez. "It can cost you your life."

Officials vowed to shut down what they said was a loosely coordinated network for recruiting patients, which they referred to as a "big business." They called in the national Centers for Disease Control and Prevention to investigate.

Notably absent from the story, however, was any comment from doctors, surgeons, or officials in the Dominican Republic, though the *Times* quoted several women from the Washington Heights area, who shrugged off the warning. One woman said she had had a $3,000 tummy tuck done in Santo Domingo a few years earlier without a problem. She told the *Times* she knew of hundreds of women from Washington Heights who had cosmetic surgery procedures done in the Dominican Republic and that only a few had complications. In fact, she said she was planning to go back again for more cosmetic surgery the next month.

NEWS GETS AROUND

The story certainly got my attention! At the time, I was in the early stages of research for this book. I was appalled. The Dominican Republic was not on my short list of countries to write about. In fact, I knew next to nothing about it. "I guess I won't be suggesting people go *there* for surgery," I said to a friend. "People will think I'm crazy."

I waited for a follow-up story that never came. No lipo-tourism sales network was closed down or even investigated; no beauty parlor operators were arrested. The story vanished from the news. It only resurfaced as a reference point anytime a reporter did a story about traveling abroad for plastic surgery.

It wasn't until a year later that I had the opportunity to personally talk to some Dominican doctors about the story, and find out that the Dominican Society of Plastic Surgery had issued a statement refuting the allegations. It never made it into *The New York Times*. The only reference I could find was reported in the Dominican Republic news. I was able to find it on a Dominican Web site:

The president of the Dominican Society of Plastic Surgery, Julio Pena Encarnacion, says that there has not been a single case of skin infection in the Dominican Republic similar to the 11 patients from New York who have lodged complaints after having operations here. The cases, which are being investigated by a team of plastic surgeons and Public Health Ministry officials, resulted in abscesses and cutaneous [skin] rashes near the area on which the surgery was performed. Pena Encarnacion said that the cause of the infection could be related to the water used, the sterilization of the instruments, or the piercings or lesions resulting from treatments carried out in beauty parlors. Yesterday, anesthesiologist Ariel Perez said the reports are due to fear of competition in the plastic surgery field in the Dominican Republic. Pena was cautious when referring to the competitive zeal as being the motive for the grievances. As reported in [the newspaper] Diario Libree, he said, "It could be a result of the competition because of the professional quality services being rendered here, but in the end, each patient opts for the physician they consider to be the most trustworthy." He mentioned that it is not only Dominicans living abroad who travel here to have surgery, but also foreigners from the United States, Puerto Rico, Curaçao, Venezuela, St. Thomas, Argentina, Switzerland, and Holland.

FACTS ARE FACTS

The costs for common cosmetic surgery procedures in the Dominican Republic are roughly 40 to 70 percent less than they are in the United States. Dominican surgeons, particularly members of the Society of Plastic Surgery, felt that they were under assault by the U.S. media, by U.S. doctors, and by U.S. politicians because of their success in attracting U.S. patients. They thought that their skill and medical facilities had been unfairly maligned.

Their suspicions were raised by the fact that their statement went unreported in *The New York Times* or anywhere in the United States and that the initial story lived on in news releases and through references in other stories. As of March 2006, the U.S. Department of State was still posting a warning on its travel advisory for the Dominican Republic:

The U.S. Embassy in Santo Domingo and the U.S. Centers for Disease Control and Prevention are aware of several cases in which U.S. citizens experienced serious complications or died following elective (cosmetic) surgery in the Dominican Republic. The CDC's Web site contains further information for all patients seeking elective surgery overseas at http://www.cdc.gov/travel/other/elective_surgery_2004.htm. Patients considering travel to the Dominican Republic for cosmetic surgery may also wish to contact the Dominican Society of Plastic Surgery (tel. 809-688-8451) to verify the training, qualifications, and reputation of specific doctors.

A similar report posted on the CDC's Web site had been taken down months before, but the scare lived on. I assumed that business for plastic surgeons in the Dominican Republic had to have gone down the tubes. Negative publicity is bad enough when it involves a single doctor but the *Times'* story was directed at the cosmetic surgeons and doctors of an entire country! What damage did it do to the country's cosmetic tourism business? Surely, I thought, it had slowed to a trickle.

Not so.

"If anything, business is better," Roberto Guerrero, M.D., of Santo Domingo told me a year after the story was published. Dr. Guerrero is a

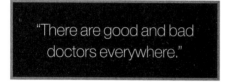

plastic surgeon who trained under Brazil's Ivo Pitanguy, M.D.; it is a credential most U.S. plastic surgeons would love to have. "People heard more about us, about what we do. If anything, the story helped us."

Dr. Guerrero, in a lengthy phone interview, defended the quality of surgery and the facilities available in the Dominican Republic. There are roughly 60 board-certified surgeons, and the requirements for certification are every bit as stringent as in the United States.

"The infections—they can happen anywhere. They happen in the U.S.," he said. "We have doctors here who are not board-certified, who do cosmetic procedures...and you have that in the U.S. as well."

But by then, Dr. Guerrero was telling me what I already knew—that there are supremely talented cosmetic and aesthetic surgeons working in the Dominican Republic in modern facilities, just as there are in Brazil, Costa Rica, Argentina, Mexico, and, of course, in the United States, and around the rest of the world. Like one woman told the *Times*: "There are good and bad doctors everywhere."

STICKS AND STONES...

On one side, we have U.S. doctors and public officials issuing a very real warning: don't go out of the country for plastic surgery, especially to the

Dominican Republic. On the other side, we have the trained medical establishment of the Dominican Republic arguing that they have been unfairly vilified for competitive reasons and with ignorance of the true state of affairs in the country. It would probably pass for journalistic fairness these days if I simply let representatives of the two views slug it out. I have certainly talked to earnest, well-spoken, successful, well-known surgeons who can do just that.

Lost in the shouting, likely, would be the common ground. I could choose a top, board-certified cosmetic surgeon in the United States and a top, board-certified surgeon in the Dominican Republic or another country and wager that they would agree on the following:

- Schooling, training, and board certification processes are substantially similar. In fact, they are so similar among the United States and other countries with modern medical schools, teaching hospitals, and national peer oversight that a discussion of the differences would only be of academic interest.
- There are similar personal standards for operating facilities, regardless of what national board is responsible for certifying the facilities.
- No patient should undergo a cosmetic procedure without fully understanding the risks and having a realistic estimation of the outcome.
- Cosmetic and aesthetic surgery should only be performed by fully trained, experienced professionals such as themselves.

It is easy to browse the World Wide Web and find successful, board-certified plastic and cosmetic surgeons with lengthy and impressive résumés and glowing recommendations from grateful patients. The only significant difference you will find among the surgeons are geographical location—and price.

Both are important factors to a patient.

The attention the don't-go-to-the-Dominican-Republic-for-cosmetic-surgery scare drew in 2004 and 2005 shows that there is controversy and confusion about medical tourism, in general, and cosmetic surgery, in particular.

The story also added credence to the notion that traveling out of the

> There is controversy and confusion about medical tourism, in general, and cosmetic surgery, in particular.

country for cosmetic surgery is a phenomenon, not an aberration. A dozen or a few dozen serious infections, while disastrous for the individual patients and alarming and confounding to their doctors, is completely unsurprising given the number of surgeries performed. In fact, one can be reasonably sure that there have been quite a few more infections than those reported and that there are many more patients who have been less than satisfied with their results.

Choosing even the best, most-experienced, and most-expensive cosmetic surgeon, whether it be in the United States or abroad, is no guarantee that a patient will heal perfectly. Certainly it must cross the minds of any person who elects to have cosmetic surgery that there is at least a small chance that he or she will be disfigured or will die. There is a somewhat greater risk that someone will simply be dissatisfied, to some degree, with the results. Top U.S. plastic surgeons complain that too much of their time is spent fixing the poor work of others from the United States and abroad. However, top surgeons in other countries make the same complaint.

The bottom line is that the Dominican Republic scare story made it manifestly clear just how price-sensitive the cosmetic surgery consumer market is. In the minds of an increasing number of consumers, the difference between a $3,000 tummy tuck overseas and a $7,000 one in the United States is, simply, $4,000; and the $4,000 represents not a cost of quality assurance but a cost some people are either unwilling or unable to bear.

The fact that the story did not hurt the cosmetic surgery business in the Dominican Republic much, if at all, says that traveling abroad for inexpensive cosmetic surgery is not a fad any more than cosmetic surgery itself is. If the price is right, Americans will shoulder some inconvenience, bear some

> Traveling abroad for cosmetic surgery is not a fad any more than cosmetic surgery itself is a fad.

uncertainty, and weigh risk when considering their medical and health-care options. They are doing it for cosmetic surgery. In lesser but growing numbers, they are doing it for other kinds of medical care, too.

AMERICAN DOCTORS SPEAK OUT

What are the real risks against which to weigh the considerable cost savings? In April of 2005, the American Society of Plastic Surgeons (ASPS) issued a briefing paper that overwhelmingly cautioned against traveling abroad for surgery, though not in the stark terms it used regarding going to the Dominican Republic. If one read nothing else, one would conclude that traveling overseas for plastic surgery is a poor idea. In the broadest context, however, the ASPS statement is full of sound advice for anyone considering cosmetic surgery. I offer the entire briefing paper, interspersed with commentary and context.

Cosmetic surgery tourism is a price-driven phenomenon that has experienced increased growth over the past decade. Numerous companies offering all-inclusive vacation packages that include cosmetic surgery are popping up all over the world and can be easily located via the Internet. The offers generally include private hospital services and tout "highly trained" and "credentialed" medical staff. Since elective cosmetic surgery procedures are not covered by insurance, price is the major selling point of cosmetic surgery tourism, with entire vacation/surgical packages costing less than individual procedures in the United States.

This is entirely true. Clearly, however, the ASPS disapproves of cosmetic surgery being a "price-driven phenomenon," even as its member surgeons continue to work on devising lower-cost, less-invasive techniques and procedures and to compete with each other. U.S. cosmetic surgeons, however, in almost all circumstances, are unable to compete on price with their counterparts in the nip-and-tuck nations of Central and South America and Asia.

Although there are many skilled and qualified physicians practicing all over (the) world, the ASPS cautions that it may be difficult to assess the training and credentials of surgeons outside of the United States. Patients may take unnecessary risks, when choosing cosmetic surgery vacations, by unknowingly selecting unqualified physicians and having procedures performed in non-accredited surgical facilities. The ASPS urges patients to consider the potential complications, unsatisfactory results, and risks to general health that may occur.

Yes, it *can* be difficult to assess the training and credentials of surgeons outside the United States. Surgeons and facilities overseas that are marketing to prospective patients in the United States, however, have made it considerably easier. Overseas surgeons offer their credentials online, and ways of verifying them are available via Internet and telephone. Prospective patients can consult directly with surgeons and staff from other countries online; references can be provided and evaluated; consultations can be conducted by phone, e-mail, Internet chat, and even via Internet video. Indeed, many ASPS members are building Internet practices in exactly this way to draw patients from around the country and from abroad.

Plastic-surgery professional organizations, no doubt, would agree whole-heartedly that the ASPS certainly can not be faulted for urging patients to consider all possible risks and to be aware of selecting unqualified physicians who operate in substandard facilities. To that I would even add a further cautionary note: People who are considering the option of going overseas for cosmetic surgery, or any other kind of health care, should keep solidly in their minds that they must be ready and willing to walk away from the decision at any point. If they come to believe they have been misled about the surgeon's expertise, the quality of the medical facility, the procedures involved, the price, or other terms, the right decision in the end may be to walk away. A patient who has done sufficient research is very unlikely to end up in such a position, but one must be mentally prepared to not go through with surgery if one develops serious doubts—even if it means cutting your losses on the expense of traveling there.

Vacation-related activities may compromise patients' health. Cosmetic surgery trips are marketed as vacations. Although enticing, vacation activities should be avoided after surgery. To properly heal and to reduce the possibility of complications, patients should not sunbathe, drink alcohol, swim/snorkel, water ski/jet ski, parasail, take extensive tours (walking or bus), or exercise after surgery.

Yes, some firms are marketing cosmetic surgery as vacation trips, and it is also true that some patients who go abroad allow for some vacation time by arriving early or extending their stays past the period of enforced recovery. Patients can certainly arrange to recover in comfortable, even luxurious, surroundings. But your surgeon abroad is going to tell you the same thing as well. Further, patients should budget extra time at the end of their trips, bearing in mind that complications and infections are possible and that you can not absolutely count on being physically ready to go home on a pre-arranged schedule.

Cosmetic surgery is real surgery. At the highest level of care, every surgery, including cosmetic surgery, has some risks. These risks may increase when procedures are performed during cosmetic surgery vacations. Infections are the most common complication seen in patients that go abroad for cosmetic surgery. Other complications include unsightly scars, hematomas, and unsatisfactory results.

Travel combined with surgery significantly increases risk of complications. Individually, long flights or surgery can increase the potential risk of developing pulmonary embolism and blood clots. Traveling combined with surgery further increases the risk of developing these potentially fatal complications, in addition to swelling and infection. Before flying, the ASPS suggests waiting five to seven days after body procedures such as liposuction and breast augmentation and seven to 10 days after cosmetic procedures of the face including facelifts, eyelid surgery, nose jobs, and laser treatments.

All good points, but it is also the same advice you would get from a qualified surgeon in any other country. Patients shouldn't ignore this advice. I don't mean to place blame, but far too many cosmetic surgery horror stories can be traced, in part, to patients not following doctor's orders for the recovery period.

Travel can be stressful and exhausting, and attempting it too soon after surgery can impede recovery. Despite the ominous tone of this caution, individual surgeons I talked to agree with this sentiment: Follow your doctor's orders if you want your best chance at a trouble-free recovery. Don't travel until your doctor says it is safe to do so.

In addition, airlines make special provisions for patients who are traveling with disabilities, and that includes travelers who have had recent surgery. If you have a long trip with flight changes, for example, it may be prudent to call the airline in advance and arrange for wheelchair service.

Follow-up care and monitoring may be limited. Follow-up care and monitoring is an important part of any surgery. Cosmetic surgery vacation packages provide limited follow-up care, if any, once the patient returns to the United States. Patients who have traveled outside of the United States for cosmetic surgery and experienced a complication may find it hard to locate a qualified plastic surgeon to treat the problem or to provide revision surgeries. Local doctors may not know what surgical techniques the physician used in the initial operation, making treatment difficult or nearly impossible. Revision surgeries can be more complicated than the initial operation and patients rarely get the desired results.

In general, this is true and should be considered carefully, especially regarding follow-up care. Some patients are afraid to tell their family doctors what they are going to do, or have already done. It's best to be as prepared as possible for complications. Many experienced patients recommend consulting with your family doctor before going overseas. Also, reputable overseas surgeons are available for consultation with you or with your doctor at home via e-mail and telephone. This is not a deal-breaker, but it is something to think about.

Bargain surgery can be costly. Patients can incur additional costs for revision surgeries and complications that may total more than the cost of the initial operation if originally performed in the United States.

Well, yes. That can happen. Bluntly, it can happen in the United States as well, and you'll be out far more money in the end. Choosing a qualified and experienced surgeon is your best chance at minimizing the risk of bad surgery that can lead to additional rounds of expensive surgery. Good cosmetic surgeons overseas often charge far less than good cosmetic surgeons in the United States. The ASPS cannot really quite get around that fact.

> Many experienced patients recommend consulting with your family doctor before going overseas.

You should ask your surgeon in advance what his or her policies are on revisions, should you be dissatisfied. Some will do revisions for free, in certain circumstances, or for a reduced charge. A cosmetic surgeon's best advertisement is satisfied customers.

Surgeon and facility qualifications may not be verifiable. In order for cosmetic surgery to be performed safely, it requires the proper administration of anesthesia, sterile technique, modern instrumentation and equipment, as well as properly trained surgeons. Vacation destinations may not have formal medical accreditation boards to certify physicians or medical facilities. Many facilities are privately owned and operated, making it difficult to check the credentials of surgeons, anesthesiologists, and other medical personnel. There are no U.S. laws that protect patients or mandate the training and qualifications of physicians who perform plastic surgery outside of the United States. There may be no legal recourse if surgical negligence by the physician or institution occurs.

If the surgeon's credentials and the quality and standards of the surgical facility can't be reasonably verified and vouched for, you shouldn't go. Simple.

As to legal remedies, should a patient be dissatisfied with surgery—or maimed or killed by it—it is true that it is easier and far more convenient to sue a U.S. doctor in the United States than it is to attempt to litigate outside our borders. However, suing a plastic surgeon in the United States is far from a slam-dunk, and reputable surgeons here and abroad are generally willing to extend themselves to produce a happy patient rather than a disgruntled one who will call a lawyer.

Devices and products used may not meet U.S. standards. Cosmetic surgery products or devices used in other countries may not have been tested, proven safe and effective, or been approved by the U.S. Food and Drug Administration (FDA). For example, an implant used in the United States must meet standards of safety and effectiveness, a process regulated by the FDA. Other countries may not have similar regulations.

Patients should, of course, check on what substances are injected and what devices are being inserted into their bodies. However, one of the reasons many American women have gone abroad for breast augmentation is the availability of silicone implants, banned by the FDA in 1992 but popular in other parts of the world. It is possible that silicone implants may again be widely available in the United States because the ASPS says silicone is safe and that the FDA should drop the ban, arguing that patients should have the option of choosing silicone. The ASPS says silicone implants are safe and the FDA, at this writing, seems inclined to allow wider testing. The ban could well be lifted at almost any time.

The ASPS briefing paper goes on to name Argentina, Brazil, Costa Rica, the Dominican Republic, Malaysia, Mexico, the Philippines, Poland, South Africa, and Thailand as cosmetic-surgery trip destinations, noting that these countries offer everything from "safari and surgery" to "tropical, scenic tour" vacation packages. It concludes with a useful checklist of questions to ask when choosing a cosmetic surgeon, clearly advocating the selection of an ASPS member. Point by point, however, the briefing paper offers advice no different than one would get from a qualified surgeon overseas—and the ASPS, though briefly, acknowledges there are many of them.

POINT, COUNTERPOINT

Rod Rohrich, M.D., a Dallas physician who is a past president of the ASPS, is perhaps the ASPS point man for the briefing paper. He reiterated many of the points in the briefing paper, stood behind them, and referred me to articles in which he had been quoted.

"People want to go for the deal. They want to go abroad because, quote unquote, 'They can get the same surgery for a reduced price.' Therein is the fallacy," is what Dr. Rohrich said in a *Fort Worth Star-Telegram* story in August 2004. "America has the best health care system in the world... You're putting yourself and your body and your life at incredible risk. Is it worth saving $500 on your face-lift if it could kill you? There are excellent surgeons in Mexico and all these countries. But I can tell you most of them don't have these fly-in, fly-out deals."

Ironically, Luiz Toledo, M.D., a surgeon in Brazil who is active in the International Society of Aesthetic Plastic Surgery (ISAPS), referred me to the same news story when I asked him for the ISAP perspective on the ASPS briefing paper. Dr. Toledo said patients generally look outside their own countries for better-quality services, cheaper prices, or a combination of the two. But he warned against seeking treatment from "cowboys"—untrained doctors with different specialties who perform cosmetic procedures for quick profits.

"A patient may travel to Brazil, Mexico, South Africa, or Costa Rica and have top-quality surgery with a cheaper price, due to the exchange rate or to economic differences between countries," Dr. Toledo said. "It is wrong, however, and it should not be encouraged to travel for surgery only because it is cheap."

It would be wrong to assume that Dr. Rohrich and Dr. Toledo have anything other than the highest respect for each other's abilities; they represent two points of view. Dr. Rohrich's is that the risks of making a bad decision in choosing an overseas surgeon,

> "It is wrong, however, and it should not be encouraged to travel for surgery only because it is cheap."

and of traveling overseas for cosmetic surgery, are simply too high. "It has nothing to do with competition," he said to me.

Dr. Toledo assesses the risks differently. In general, I have found that medical professionals do not want to make statements that mark them as at odds with their professional associations, associates, or peers. At the same time, it would be a mistake to think that the briefing paper is representative of all opinions on the subject of medical tourism within the ASPS.

THE BEST OF BOTH WORLDS

John J. Corey, M.D., a prominent plastic surgeon in Scottsdale, Arizona, is an ASPS member. However, he also advertises a Brazilian influence on his practice and his technique; Dr. Corey traveled to Brazil in 1993 and studied under the aforementioned Ivo Pitanguy, M.D.

"Brazilian surgeons seem to have a different 'eye' for aesthetic surgery...a different way of analyzing beauty and the human form. We Americans have a tendency to be very technical. We want to know exactly how much to contour and how much to measure. Brazilians seem to approach procedures more artistically. They don't rely on applying the same measurement to every woman. They really believe in sculpting the form and creating the curves and lines of the feminine shape."

Dr. Corey doesn't deny the obvious implication of his own words—that many Brazilian surgeons are incredibly good and that U.S. surgeons can and do learn a lot from them. And, like many other surgeons in the United States and abroad, he has used the Internet in building and extending his own practice. He has patients from out of state and out of the country. He also knows that not all patients can afford his prices, and that excellent surgeons, board-certified in Brazil and other countries, charge far less than he does in Scottsdale.

> Brazilians approach procedures more artistically. They believe in sculpting the form and creating the curves and lines of the female shape.

"The ASPS is going to come down on the side of caution and safety," Dr. Corey said. "And I don't think anyone can fault them for doing that; it is what doctors do. But at the same time, of course, there are well-qualified surgeons around the world. We interact with each other; we learn from each other. And economic conditions, and the cost of doing business, are different in other countries."

Dr. Corey looks at medical tourism from a pragmatic point of view. "I think we have to look at more ways to cooperate, more ways in which we can serve patients better," he suggested. "Clearly, overseas surgeons who are able to charge less are meeting a need in the market, and the market is evolving. There are ways in which doctors in the United States can be part of that, and in which patients will benefit." The ASPS, he points out, does list on its Web site "corresponding members" from overseas; there are not that many surgeons who have chosen to affiliate, however, and the ASPS notes that it can not vouch for their credentials.

> American doctors are going to come down on the side of caution and safety. This is what doctors do.

IF YOU CAN'T BEAT THEM...

Oscar Suárez, M.D., is head of the Department of Plastic Surgery at CIMA Hospital in San José, Costa Rica. CIMA is a modern, private facility where a number of Costa Rican surgeons cater primarily to patients from the United States.

"The surgeons in the United States., the ones I talk to, are of two minds about medical tourism," Dr. Suárez said in an interview. "Some are against it. And others, they want to be part of it." Dr. Suárez said he has been contacted by a number of peers in the United States who are interested in partnerships or opening facilities in Costa Rica.

That a patient can find experienced and talented cosmetic and aesthetic surgeons in a number of countries around the world is not a matter in serious dispute. Surgeons can disagree as to the risks involved in traveling and as to the difficulty of choosing a good surgeon. In the end, however, those are considerations for individual patients to weigh. Prominent, qualified, and experienced surgeons from all countries emphatically counsel patients that they should not choose a surgeon based on price alone.

PRICES IN THE UNITED STATES AND ABROAD

Consumers who consider going abroad to save money for cosmetic surgery, dental work, or any other kind of medical care, will hear these bromides, either from voices in their heads or from well-meaning friends and relatives:

You get what you pay for.

If it sounds too good to be true, it probably is.

Quality doesn't come cheap.

One does not have to have an intimate knowledge of international economics to understand why prices for high-quality cosmetic surgery can be far lower in less-developed countries than in the United States or Western Europe. A good surgeon is an artist, a psychologist, and modern-day wizard of sorts who transforms and restores; but he or she is also a businessperson. Cosmetic surgeons treat patients and are paid fees; cosmetic surgeons whose services are in demand can and do charge higher fees.

Simple, right? You get what you pay for, and quality doesn't come cheap. However, among other things, geography matters a great deal. In your own town or city, you may find a range of prices from different cosmetic surgeons, as you might expect. Well-known surgeons with years of experience and hundreds or even thousands of satisfied customers will charge the most. A surgeon fresh from his or her residency, just starting out, trained but relatively inexperienced, will charge less. It is not unheard of for surgeons just starting out to offer reduced fees to clients who will agree to provide testimonials or referrals or otherwise participate in marketing the new business.

In your town, there will also be doctors and surgeons who may not be board certified in plastic surgery who nonetheless legally practice it, to an extent. The ASPS warns that such practitioners may be less-safe choices and, generally speaking, one would guess that they are right. Still, it goes on.

The average price of a typical face-lift in the United States performed by a board-certified plastic surgeon in an accredited surgical facility, including surgeon's fee, anesthesia fee, and operating facility fee, is in the $7,000 to $9,000 range, according to InfoPlasticSurgery.com That might be the range in your town. But if you live in New York City, the range might be 50 percent higher. If you live in parts of the less-urban South or Midwest, the range might be a little lower. Geography matters, even within the United States. There is more demand for cosmetic and aesthetic surgery and procedures in urban areas and on the coasts; and the costs of living and of doing business are correspondingly higher.

So how can board-certified, experienced surgeons working in modern facilities in Mexico, Brazil, Costa Rica, the Dominican Republic, Thailand, India, and other countries charge so much less? While a face-lift abroad is more likely to cost between $3,500 and $6,000, including travel, meals, and accommodations, the costs of living and of doing business is correspondingly less in these countries. The top surgeons in the world, those with international reputations, can charge and get U.S. prices wherever they may be, but the many trained and qualified surgeons who aspire to be known as among the elite in the world must charge far less to draw patients from abroad, including the United States. And they can make a good living doing so.

Many think U.S. surgeons are greedy, but I do not think that is the case. They face significantly higher costs than do their counterparts and peers in other countries. In many ways, the reasons prices for cosmetic and other surgeries are lower in other countries than in the United States and Western Europe are the same reasons why it is less expensive to produce DVD players or textiles abroad: They have less-expensive land, less-expensive construction costs, lower labor costs, lower taxes, and lower administrative costs. It is a mistake to single out any one thing as being responsible for the difference.

Malpractice insurance costs are also partly to blame. Though malpractice rates vary, depending on amounts of coverage, U.S. surgeons I interviewed said they each pay between $40,000 and $70,000 annually, compared to the less than $6,000 a year a Brazilian surgeon I know pays. This is a substantial difference, yet a small part of the overall equation. About the only business expense that is the same for surgeons regardless of where they live is medical equipment and medical supplies.

Price is relative from country to country, and a patient looking at the possibility of traveling abroad for care can responsibly factor that in.

> Prices are relative from country to country; some prices are so low that one should be suspicious.

Some prices are so low that one can not help but be suspicious. Substantial inquiries are merited and references should be required. Cosmetic and elective surgery prices in the Far East are, for the most part, somewhat lower than those in South America, which are somewhat lower than those in Central America. I know that there are good surgeons in all those places.

Surgeons in the Far East, in fact, may be more likely to have trained in the United States and be fluent in English, though they have no monopoly on either of those things.

The cosmetic surgeon who charges the highest prices in your town may well be among the best and will almost certainly be among the most experienced. But paying the highest price does not guarantee the best outcome. Is a $10,000 face-lift in New York City better than a $7,000 one in Cincinnati? Is either better than a $3,000 one in Brazil? It depends.

I have talked to people who are unhappy with their expensive cosmetic work and people who are thrilled with the quality of their inexpensive results. For every anecdote, there is another one to give lie to the first. Beyond the borders of the United States, options abound for those willing to take the time to investigate, analyze, and choose.

In discussing medical tourism with people in the United States who are only casually acquainted with the subject, I am perhaps most often asked, "But wouldn't I be better off choosing a doctor from the United States?" My best answer evolved over time: Someone is probably better off choosing a doctor from the United States if he or she is simply picking a doctor or surgeon at random. If you are going to leave your decision essentially to chance—say with no more help than a phone book or HMO directory—you are probably best off staying close to home. But if you are going to research your choice and compare and contrast doctors, surgeons, and medical facilities—your options expand dramatically. Like the woman told *The New York Times*, "there are good doctors and bad doctors everywhere."

CHAPTER 3

A Brief and Selective History of Medical Tourism

My dear Athos,

*I wish, as your health absolutely requires it, that you should rest for a
fortnight. Go, then, and take the waters of Forges, or any that may be
more agreeable to you, and recuperate yourself as quickly as possible.*

Your affectionate,
de Treville

—The Three Musketeers
Alexandre Dumas, 1844

The history of cosmetic surgery—and of traveling extended distances
for medical care or health reasons—goes back to the beginning of
recorded time. Reconstructive plastic surgery procedures were
performed in India at least as far back as 600 B.C.[1]

Literature and history are replete with stories of people who have traveled for health reasons—the healing and recuperative powers of bathing
in the hot mineral springs around the world is documented in both fact
and in fiction. School children are taught that the Spanish explorer Ponce
de Leon allegedly went in search of the Fountain of Youth and found
Florida and death by an Indian arrow instead. I say "allegedly" because a
number of scholars dismiss the Fountain of Youth part of the story as
myth. In more recent history, Franklin D. Roosevelt received therapeutic
baths and muscle treatments for his debilitating pain from polio in Warm
Spring, Colorado during his administration from 1933 to 1945, making the
place sort of a western White House for months at a time.

You could say that President Roosevelt was a pioneer of modern health
tourism, the precursor of medical tourism, though the two are distinct,
historically and even today. Health tourism is the business of spas selling
weekend or week-long indulgences of luxurious massages, exotic baths,

healthy foods, beauty makeovers, and soothing or exhilarating scenery for an even more exhilarating price. Some even have a spiritual component. The actual medicinal value of much of this has long been debated, though many medical professionals vouch for its therapeutic benefits.

Medical tourism, on the other hand, is entirely recent and has become the more narrowly applied term for traveling abroad for the services of a doctor or surgeon. Recuperating in a spa or vacation-like setting is an option, and an attractive embellishment for many. While, no doubt, there are scholars who could step forward with examples from history of people who traveled great distances for the services of a particular doctor or a particular treatment or surgery, they would also acknowledge that medical tourism is mostly a modern phenomenon. It tracks very closely with the 20th-century refinement of cosmetic surgery as a medical specialty spawned from necessity during World War I when reconstructive techniques were developed to treat those maimed in combat.

> Recuperating in a spa or vacation-like setting is an option, and an attractive embellishment for many.

By the 1950s, the groundwork for what was to become modern cosmetic surgery had been laid. Though far from common, surgery for purely aesthetic reasons had become less peculiar. Initially there was little competition. Through the 1950s and 1960s, cosmetic surgery was the province of the United States and Europe; the clients, whatever nationality, were mostly wealthy. Quick, affordable international air travel was the first precondition for medical tourism to emerge and international patients started to head for the great hospitals of the United States and Europe, as they still do today. The main difference today is that the international competition to provide medical services has become fierce.

In addition to the patients, however, an ever-increasing number of medical students, doctors, and surgeons from around the world converged on the United States and Europe seeking medical training. As time passed, more information was exchanged and spread; more technology was shared. Some of the medical students stayed in the United

States as part of the infamous "brain drain" that was attracting the best and the brightest from around the world, to the detriment of efforts to modernize and improve economic conditions abroad. But some went home to build medical practices in their own countries and to found new institutes, hospitals, and centers of learning. Among the skills they took with them were cosmetic surgery techniques.

In time, inevitably, other destinations for patients besides the United States and Europe arose.

THE PIONEERS

Brazil, in particular, gradually became known internationally for the expertise of its aesthetic and plastic surgeons, but it was not a fame that extended to the mass consumer markets of the more economically developed world. Prof. Dr. Ivo Pitanguy is not a household name outside of his home country, where he is revered. Dr. Pitanguy has performed or guided thousands of surgeries in a storied, five-decade career and has trained more than 500 plastic surgeons from more than 40 countries who practice internationally, making cosmetic surgery expertise and technique one of Brazil's best-known exports.

Among his peers, Dr. Pitanguy is the father of modern cosmetic surgery. He also has become the father of modern medical tourism, for those he has trained are among the most sought after surgeons in the world. Yet his name and his work, outside Brazil and South America, are familiar primarily only to other plastic surgeons, Brazilians living abroad, and the families and friends of his patients—not to the millions of potential plastic surgery patients in the United States who are far more likely to know the names of surgeons on *Dr. 90210* or *The Swan*.

In the United States, if one had to name a doctor who was famous in international medicine during the 1960s, perhaps the only household name was Christiaan Barnard, M.D., the South African who performed the world's first heart transplant in 1967. Notably, Dr. Barnard trained in the United States, as did Dr. Pitanguy, before heading home to eventual renown.

I cite Dr. Pitanguy and Dr. Barnard as pioneers not so much for their unquestioned skill as surgeons but because they achieved the kind of international fame that, for most of the 20th century, was reserved for doctors and scientists only in the West (North America and Western Europe) and, to a lesser degree, the East (mostly the former Soviet Union). Patients in Eastern bloc countries frequently traveled to the then-USSR and its allied nations for advanced medical care. For all of the 20th century, and even into the beginning of the 21st century, the vast majority of medical tourists were not jetting to South America or Africa, let alone the Far or Middle East. They were coming to the world's great doctors and hospitals in the United States and in Europe.

From the perspective of the United States, in particular, this state of affairs served, and still serves, to reinforce the generally held belief that the United States has the finest medical care in the world. In the last 50 years, only Dr. Barnard's achievement challenged this notion in the popular imagination. People were oddly comforted when Drs. Denton Cooley and Michael DeBakey started transplanting hearts in Houston, Texas, almost in the same way they were when the United States finally answered the Soviet space challenge of Sputnik.

Meanwhile, Dr. Pitanguy just kept doing what he was doing. Patients spread the word. Brazil was and is the mecca of plastic and cosmetic surgery, challenged only recently by Southern California. The surgeons Dr. Pitanguy trained spread out through South and Central America and around the world. Over time, a second essential precondition for medical tourism to emerge as big business was met—medical talent spread out, belonging less exclusively to the developed world. In economically emerging nations, improving health care was a

> Brazil was and is the mecca of plastic and cosmetic surgery, challenged only recently by southern California.

priority—which meant building more modern medical facilities. The quality of care in the less-developed world rose steadily, at least in metropolitan areas, but prices for medical services remained low, relative to the United States and Europe.

BUILD IT, AND THEY WILL COME

Arnoldo Fournier, M.D., a cosmetic surgeon in San José, Costa Rica, was one of the pioneers in marketing his services abroad. He came to Costa Rica in the early 1980s, fresh from his residency at St. Luke's Hospital in New York, and was told that there was no demand for aesthetic procedures in Costa Rica. Stubbornly, he stayed and went after the U.S. market. He placed his first ad in the *Tico Times*, the Central American country's English-language daily; later, he turned to the flight magazines of the international airlines: *LACSA, Eastern, Skyward,* and *Passages* among them.

By the 1990s, Dr. Fournier and other Costa Rican cosmetic surgeons, dentists, and doctors thought they had a pretty good thing going. Costa Rica was beginning to prosper as a tourist destination and U.S. retirees were

> Costa Rica began to prosper as a medical tourist destination in the 1990s— about the same time as increasing numbers of U.S. retirees were making the country their home.

making the country their home in increasing numbers; the number of Americans desiring cosmetic surgery was starting to rachet up.

Prices for cosmetic surgery in Costa Rica then, as now, were much lower than in the United States. I received an e-mail in December of 2004 from a woman in Florida who had read what I had written about my own trip for dental work; she affectionately recalled going to see my dentist, "Dr. Telma," in 1986. She wrote:

> *In 1986, Dr. Telma installed 13 crowns in my mouth for $1,200. At that time, if I had this work performed in the U.S., it would have cost about $4,000 to $6,000…As she worked, Dr. Telma and I also had incredible intellectual discussions on the anthropology of Central American Indians, their bone structure and diet, and where they came from. Both she and her husband are very well educated in many other areas, and not just dentistry…I came across your article as I was searching the 'net for her services again. I need two crowns and some teeth bleaching, and a minor face lift, which I am going to coordinate and schedule this summer if possible.*

So what was to become known later as medical tourism was already growing in Costa Rica in the 1980s and into the 1990s. In what was to prove to be a prescient report, the World Bank in September 1995 published a 52-page study on *Prospects for Health Tourism Exports for the English-Speaking Caribbean.*[2] It noted:

> *Direct patient care is the major health service exported by Costa Rica. In addition to plastic surgery, a full range of pediatric and adult services including high technology dependent procedures such as open heart surgery are exported.*
>
> *Costa Rica's target markets for the export of health services are the United States, other Central American countries, Puerto Rico, Barbados, and other Caribbean nations, Colombia, Venezuela, Canada, and Spain.*

The prescient part of the study identified the reasons why potential for further substantial growth existed in the Caribbean countries:

- **Demographics in target markets** (for example, aging post-war baby boomers who are concerned about physical appearance, semi-retirement, full retirement and relaxation) will mean marked increases in demand for cosmetic surgery, spas, and retirement communities.
- **The growing affluent class of baby boomers** may be less price sensitive and more sensitive to other aspects of the marketing mix (for example, location and confidentiality).
- **Lifestyles in Europe and North America** increase the demand for services such as spas, fitness centers, cosmetic work, or addiction treatment centers.
- **Waiting time for procedures** in the United Kingdom and, to a lesser extent, in Canada encourages the search for outside health services.
- **A large portion of the U.S. population is uninsured or underinsured.**
- **Private insurance does not cover selected treatments.**
- **Operations in Caribbean regions appeal to doctors** from target markets that enjoy visiting the region, which could facilitate strategic alliances and capital investment.

- **Lifestyle health-related problems in the target markets** are similar to those among people in the Caribbean, and quality health and social marketing materials could be exported to these markets.

The report stated:

The U.S. market is most apt to offer opportunities to the Caribbean because it has a large uninsured and underinsured population, it has very high prices, and it is geographically close to the Caribbean. Moreover, the U.S. system is more fragmented and less controlled than health sectors in other industrialized countries. As a result, the U.S. market has multiple avenues of entry.

The report also summed up the challenges facing countries going after the health tourism market as well, among them that:

- U.S. medical doctors act as "gatekeepers" for the U.S. health-care system and would not want to lose patients to the Caribbean market.
- Questions about quality of care in the Caribbean will exist in consumers' minds and will be difficult to overcome.
- Neighboring countries in Latin America could provide care at lower cost, as could countries in Eastern Europe.

Other than leaving out the entry of Asian, Middle Eastern, or African nations into the market, the World Bank study was a blueprint for medical tourism for the next decade for anyone who cared to follow it. However, it made no particular impact then that I can discover now. What it stated was already obvious to pioneers in Costa Rica and elsewhere, but it took years for much of the world to begin to notice.

The third and final precondition for medical tourism to become a globe-straddling business was that people had to know about it; it had to be marketed to a broader audience, somehow. The Internet came along at just about the right time.

Dr. Fournier claims he was the seventh cosmetic surgeon in the world to put up a Web site and I have no reason to doubt him; whether he was 7th or 17th, or 70th doesn't matter much. U.S. cosmetic surgeons were quick to seize on the new medium of Internet marketing to spread information and awareness, but several of the Costa Ricans were right there with them, as were surgeons in other countries. Once reliant for marketing solely on word of mouth, occasional visits to the United States, and flight magazines, cosmetic surgeons around the world found they had a platform from which they could reach customers directly and at a minimal cost. As the demand for cosmetic surgery in the world's No. 1 market, the United States, shifted into overdrive in the late 1990s, more surgeons abroad targeted the U.S. Though their market share was tiny, their growth rate likely was faster than that in the U.S., and it remains so today. Business for foreign surgeons in 2005 was threefold, or fivefold (depending on who you ask) what it was in 1995, when it was already going well.

Around 1998, the phrase "medical tourism" finally began creeping into news accounts. *The Washington Times* noted in March of 1998 that medical tourism was one of the few bright spots in the economy of Castro's Cuba. In April, officials in Miami, Florida were touting "the concept of medical tourism" in an Associated Press article. They

> As the demand for cosmetic surgery shifted into overdrive in the U.S., more surgeons from abroad targeted the U.S. market.

were not talking about patients going abroad or even coming from abroad; the Miami Health Care Alliance simply thought maybe vacationers who were coming to Florida might like to visit a few doctors, seeing as how they were in town anyway. If you look in a big database of periodicals and magazines published prior to 2001, most of the references to medical tourism come from overseas. The *New Straits Times* of Malaysia ran a number of stories about the potential of medical tourism for that country, for India, and for the rest of the Pacific Rim nations. The *Jerusalem Post* in 1999 referred to medical tourism as "a huge business." But if it was a huge business, it was a remarkably unreported one in the United States in the late 1990s. For me, the earliest reference to medical

tourism that bestowed proper global context to the term belonged to Prof.
Sander Gilman, author of *Making the Body Beautiful: A Cultural History of
Aesthetic Surgery*. He wrote:

> *The globalization of aesthetic surgery has spawned numerous centers
> that link surgery and tourism. North Americans have long gone to
> Mexico, the Dominican Republic, and Brazil; now the United Kingdom
> has started to offer "aesthetic surgery" tours for Americans as well.
> People in the United Kingdom flock to Marbella in Spain for discreet
> face-lifts, but Poland and Russia are now competing for this market. For
> medical tourists in the Middle East, Israel has become the country of
> choice for many procedures, even for citizens of countries that do not
> have political ties to Israel; Germans visit South Africa for breast reduc-
> tions and penis enlargements as well as to see the Kruger National
> Park; South Korea and Singapore are important for the Asian market;
> and Beirut, Lebanon, is the place to go for quick, no-questions-asked
> transgender surgery. Medical tourism has become big business, and
> aesthetic surgery, because of its elective nature, is a large part of the
> action. For every procedure recorded in one country, similar procedures
> are being undertaken on that country's citizens elsewhere...Aesthetic
> surgery has become a worldwide phenomenon in the past few decades.*

THE MEDIA IMPRIMATUR

The media in the United States did not really discover medical tourism
until 2004-05, and it was found in the Far East rather than in central and
South America. It was **Bumrungrad Hospital in Thailand** and the **Apollo
Hospitals Group in India** and **Penang Adventist Hospital in Malaysia** that
made *60 Minutes* and the front pages of the *Wall Street Journal* and *The
New York Times*, not the plucky surgeons and dentists of Costa Rica,
Mexico, and Brazil—even though far more U.S. citizens were heading
south for inexpensive medical and dental care and surgery than were
heading to the Far East. There are a few good reasons for that, which I
offer not as an apology for the media but as explanation:

1. The story wasn't about cosmetic surgery, which, despite its popularity and the professionalism of its practitioners, doesn't get the same treatment in the news as does "real" medicine. Cosmetic surgery news is fluffier, more frivolous, than open-heart surgery news. The international hospitals of the Far East, wisely, didn't play up cosmetic surgery—though they do a lot of it. They played up cardiothoracic surgery, and their state-of-the-art technology and facilities, and thus were taken more seriously. For the first time, much was made of the fact that there are an estimated 42 million people in the United States who lack adequate medical insurance who could go out of the country to get treatment they could not otherwise afford.

2. The story was delivered in part as a business story with big dollar signs, the kind that gets attention from the media. India put a $2 billion sticker on medical tourism. As previously noted, Bumrungrad sees more than 350,000 patients a year.

3. The story was generated by big multipurpose hospitals, and supported by the tourism and economic development officials of their respective countries. This is the way countries in the Far East go after markets, and there is nothing in Central or South America to compare as yet.

As we move through the first decade of the 21st century, medical tourism is still both newly discovered and in transition. The tip of the iceberg remains elective medical care, mostly cosmetic surgery and dentistry; beneath the surface is the larger consumer health-care market of the United States and Europe.

And the press is paying attention. In February 2006 a West Virginia state leglislator introduced the first bill in the country providing for the outsourcing of medical care to foreign countries. In Chicago, Blue Cross/Blue Shield investigated and then approved payment for an uninsured child's heart surgery in India. And when President Bush visited India for the first time in March 2006, the two countries released a statement pledging American support for Indian efforts to promote medical tourism, saying there is "enormous potential for collaboration" in health tourism.

Notes

1   NatiRana RE, Arora BS. History of plastic surgery in India. J Postgrad Med 2002;48:76-8.

2   Maggie Huff-Rousselle et al. *Prospects for Health Tourism Exports for the English-Speaking Caribbean.* Sept. 1995.

3   Sander L. Gilman, *Making the Body Beautiful: A Cultural History of Aesthetic Surgery.* Princeton University Press, 2001, 8.

CHAPTER 4

You're Going
Abroad for ...
What!?

In more than a year of travel, interviewing, and reading, I have run across but one example of a medical procedure for which demand has declined overseas because prices in the United States became more competitive.

"We don't do so many hair transplants as we used to," commented Joseph Cohen, M.D., sitting in his office at the Rosenstock-Lieberman Center for Cosmetic Plastic Surgery in San José, Costa Rica. "The price came down in the States; there is not so much of a difference anymore. So people don't come to us for that as much."

Dr. Cohen, who did his undergraduate work in California and his residency in general surgery in Pennsylvania, also told me that if he needed heart surgery, he would prefer to be in one of the top hospitals in the United States. Not that there are not fine heart surgeons in Costa Rica; but he would have a preference for the United States. "They have the most experience and that's what you want," he said.

What procedures do people go overseas for, and why?

As of now, inexpensive cosmetic surgery and dentistry is the leading edge of medical tourism, at least as far as North Americans and Europeans are concerned. Weight loss surgery (WLS) of various kinds for the morbidly obese is also gaining in popularity, though some insurance plans in the United States provide coverage for that. Patients go abroad for every conceivable kind of medical care if the cost savings justifies the inconvenience and any perceived risk.

Of course, patients who are covered by insurance in the United States elect to have their surgeries and procedures done in the United States for the obvious reason that they will no longer be saving money by going outside of the country. However, there are exceptions. In some cases, patients prefer going out of the country because a foreign doctor or surgeon is renowned for his or her expertise in a particular procedure. Insurance companies, includings HMOs, have been known in certain cases to treat out-of-country care no differently than they treat out-of-network care in the United States. But this is something you need to check beforehand.

A more general exception is dental work. Most dental insurance plans in the United States effectively exclude major cosmetic work, either by way of defining what is covered, or effectively, by capping the amount of coverage annually or by procedure. Insured dental patients may have some minimal reimbursement difference to factor into their decision as to whether to go abroad or not, but in the case of major work—implants or full-mouth reconstruction—the savings for going overseas remains substantial and a compelling reason to consider it as an option.

> Insurance companies have been known to treat out-of-country care no differently than they treat out-of-network care.

In general, plastic surgeons in all countries perform a variety of procedures and services. Botox, facial "fillers" for wrinkles, lip augmentation, permanent makeup, and the like are all available around the world and are generally less expensive than in the United States. Many patients who go out of the country for more costly procedures will have additional procedures done on the trip as well, but it makes little sense to go to the expense of traveling if one is only seeking relatively low-cost, non-invasive procedures.

This chapter offers a rundown of some of the more common elective procedures for which people are willing to travel overseas to save money. Be forewarned that the prices cited are estimations and, depending on the surgeon, place, and time, can be more or even less than the ranges given. I attempted to be both cautious and reasonable in checking costs.

Prospective patients should remember that surgeons have varying prices for many reasons and that important among those reasons are experience and reputation for quality. Surgeons in less-developed countries generally have a lower price structure overall because their costs are substantially lower than those in the United States or Western Europe.

Another important consideration within the following summary is that not all surgeons define the same procedures exactly the same way. A

face-lift to one may be just the centerpiece of several procedures, each
with a price that may be necessary to achieve the patient's desired result
(for example, face-lift, plus facial liposuction, neck or chin lift and work),
while another may include several procedures as part of "just a face-lift."
Also, some surgeons will offer discounts for patients who undergo multiple procedures at the same time, as in so-called extreme makeovers.

When considering prices, prospective patients have to figure out and
factor in all travel costs, which
can also vary substantially.

For my own part, I did not
choose the least-expensive dentists in the world, or even in Costa
Rica. I first satisfied myself as to
the quality of care I would receive

> Surgeons have varying
> prices for many reasons,
> experience and reputation
> for quality among them.

from a particular dentist. I could have "shopped" more extensively but
decided against it in the end. I knew that my savings would be substantial
when measured against what I could expect to pay in the United States,
and that was good enough for me. I saved at least $10,000, and perhaps I
could have saved more; but I was comfortable with my choice.

COSMETIC SURGERIES AND PROCEDURES

There are new cosmetic techniques and new variations of old ones being
tested and tried all the time by creative and innovative surgeons around
the world. Below are some of the most common ones, with their general
definitions, some tips and advice gleaned from patients and surgeons,
and some general price comparison information. Price ranges are rough
measures; the figures I use here represent approximations based on a
number of sources. You can almost certainly find surgeons in both the
United States and abroad who charge less than the lowest figures I cite,
and you can absolutely find surgeons who charge and get higher prices
for their work.

There is far more information available online, of course. How to go about
researching surgical information on the Internet is covered in chapter 5.

Liposuction/Lipoplasty

Liposuction is a procedure that can help **sculpt the body by removing unwanted fat from specific areas, including the abdomen, hips, buttocks, thighs, knees, upper arms, chin, cheeks, and neck**. Good plastic surgeons are generally fastidious about reminding patients that cosmetic surgery is "real surgery," and this is particularly true of liposuction. "Getting a little lipo" should not be trivialized. Experienced cosmetic surgeons wince at the suggestion that liposuction is easy and cringe at the thought of a cannula (the fat-suctioning tool) in unpracticed hands.

Liposuction is both physically demanding work and an art, according to its leading practitioners. Improvements in technique over the past decade have brought into use the term liposculpture, emphasizing both that the procedure is an art and that surgeons can be remarkably precise, even restoring fat to some areas to achieve the desired result.

Patients often ask about "aggressive" liposuction; in general, liposuction is for removal of relatively small volumes of fat that resist dieting and exercise. Some surgeons—including experienced ones both in the United States and abroad—will go beyond that, but one should not assume that more is better. More can be riskier; more will also involve a lengthier convalescence and recovery.

> Good plastic surgeons are fastidious about reminding patients that cosmetic surgery is "real surgery."

Liposuction is generally priced by the number of areas from which a patient wants fat removed in a session, with discounts offered for additional areas beyond the first. Prices in the United States can range from around $2,500 to $5,000 for a single area on up to more than $10,000 for five areas. The range is much lower overseas but again depends on the need of the individual patient. My guesstimate, looking at prices in Central and South America and Asia, is that median prices are 40 to 75 percent less than in the United States, or about $1,000 to $3,000 and more for up to five areas.

Face-lift (Rhytidectomy)

A face-lift is a **highly individualized procedure and is often done in conjunction with other facial procedures**. Surgeons these days strive for a natural appearance. Gone is the pulled-back, stretched look more common a generation ago. **A basic face-lift does not eliminate wrinkles**. It does not directly address the forehead area or upper eyes. It does generally address the neck area. A neck lift is usually part of a face-lift but some surgeons will do it separately.

Surgeons can recommend newer, less-invasive or noninvasive (and less expensive) alternatives to a full face-lift. My feeling about new facial surgical techniques is that there is an increased amount of uncertainty as to results and that patients should be extra-cautious until the techniques are proven.

The average cost of a face-lift in the United States is in the range of $7,000 to $10,000, but adding in other facial procedures can easily double the bill. Again, the price overseas is generally 40 to 75 percent less. A facelift in Brazil or Costa Rica can run in the $2,500 to $3,500 range.

Eyelids (Blepharoplasty)

Eyelid surgery is a procedure to **remove fat—usually along with excess skin and muscle—from the upper and lower eyelids**. Eyelid surgery can correct drooping upper lids, and puffiness or bags below the eyes.

Upper and lower eyelid work will cost $4,000 to $6,000, on average, in the United States. Once again, in examining the Web sites of reputable and experienced surgeons overseas and in researching, one will find a range of perhaps $1,300 to $2,200.

Forehead/Brow Lift

A forehead lift **can raise the eyebrows to a higher and more (presumably) aesthetic position**. It should also improve lateral hoods (the droopy flaps of skin that hang over the outside corners of the eyes.) A forehead lift should also soften horizontal forehead wrinkles and lines between the eyebrows.

A forehead lift in the United States costs in the range of about $3,500 to $5,000. The average cost abroad falls into the $1,300 to $2,000 range.

Nose Reshaping (Rhinoplasty)

Reshaping the nose is considered by many plastic surgeons to **be one of the most delicate and difficult aesthetic procedures**.

Prices can vary substantially depending on what the patient wants. A rhinoplasty can cost from $5,000 to $8,000 or more in the United States. In general, median prices abroad, however, are 40 to 75 percent less than in the United States, or from about $1,250 to $6,000.

Chemical Peels (light, medium, deep)

A chemical peel is aimed at **destroying outer layers of old skin, inducing the growth of new skin**. The lightest of peels may be inexpensive ($50 to $100, even in the United States) and part of some regular beauty regimens. In many states, a medical degree is not required to administer even heavier chemical peels. Having seen people who had deep chemical peels, I for one can only barely imagine allowing a doctor, let alone anyone with lesser training, to do this to me. For days after a deep chemical peel, it's difficult for someone who has never seen one before to think that they will ever look normal again. But the final results can be extraordinary.

Deep chemical peels in the U.S. can cost $1,500 to $2,500; overseas, they can cost from $300 to $800.

Breast Lift (Mastopexy)

A breast lift, or mastopexy, **is a surgical procedure to raise and reshape sagging breasts** by removing excess skin and repositioning the remaining tissue and nipples. The price in the U.S. is in the range of $4,000 to $6,000; abroad it can be $1,200 to $2,500. Breast reduction, if desired, can be encompassed in this procedure. It may or may not cost more, depending on the individual and the surgeon.

Breast Augmentation

Increasing breast size by means of **surgical implants remains controversial, particularly in the United States, but they nevertheless have soared in popularity**, even after silicone implants were mostly banned in the United States in 1992. Only saline implants have been in widespread use in the United States since then, though the U.S. Food and Drug Administration, which regulates the types of implants allowed, relaxed restrictions in 2005.

Silicone implants have never been banned overseas and their supporters say the products have been improved and made safer over the years. There seems little doubt that many American women have gone abroad for breast augmentation surgery not just because it is 40 to 75 percent less expensive but also because they have wanted the firmer and more realistic silicone gel implants. Costs in the United States generally range from about $5,000 to $8,000 and up; the overseas cost is in the $2,000 to $4,000 range.

Arm Lift (Brachioplasty)

An arm lift is a procedure to **remove loose skin and excess fat deposits in the upper arm**. The procedure is most commonly desired by patients who have lost significant weight, leaving them with loose skin in the upper arms. U.S. costs are in the $5,000 to $7,000 range. Overseas, the price range goes from about $1,500 to $4,000.

Tummy Tuck (Abdominoplasty)

A tummy tuck is a major surgical procedure to **remove excess skin and fat from the middle and lower abdomen and to tighten the muscles of the abdominal wall**. The procedure is often combined with liposuction and, done properly, it can more or less eliminate the unwanted flab and loose skin that result from pregnancy. A tummy tuck in the United States can cost $5,000 to $9,000; a tummy tuck abroad can run from $1,500 to $3,500 or so.

Perhaps even more so than with other surgeries and procedures, patients who have a tummy tuck done abroad will need to consider how much recovery time they will need before being able to travel. It is also important that they follow their doctor's orders regarding recovery. The immediate effect is often disabling; patients may be unable to work for two to four weeks, and may have restricted physical activity longer than that.

Anecdotally, I have heard more about complications from tummy tucks and breast augmentations than I have heard of problems resulting from all other plastic surgeries combined—and, often, the stories come with the patient's confession: "I know I tried to do too much, too soon."

Surgeons can also do "mini tummy tucks" that do not include as much muscle repair and tightening. Tummy tucks can be highly personalized surgeries (as are most major cosmetic procedures.) The procedure is both less invasive and less expensive; surgeons caution that the results are not as emphatic as with a full procedure. The cost in the United States can range from $1,800 to $6,000. The cost abroad can be from $1,200 to $3,000.

Lower Body Lift (Belt Lipectomy)

A lower body lift **removes excess tissue from the lateral hip and inner thigh**, addressing sagging skin resulting from aging, pregnancy, or extreme weight fluctuations. It is often performed in combination with liposuction and a tummy tuck and other procedures, which makes pricing a highly individual matter.

Lower body lifts are frequently **part of so-called "extreme makeovers" for people who have lost large amounts of weight**, either through diet and exercise or as a result of weight loss (bariatric) surgery. While insurance may cover weight loss surgery, I have yet to hear of an insurer that covers the cosmetic surgery many patients feel is necessary after losing 150 pounds or more.

Such patients may want a range of procedures that can cost $20,000 to $50,000 and more in the United States. The price range abroad can be more like $8,000 to $15,000. Patients having such extensive surgery abroad must be prepared to be away from home for at least a month, or to make more than one trip. There are various procedures that are less drastic, including procedures that address only the buttocks, lower back, and/or upper thighs.

Buttocks Implants (Gluteal Augmentation)

Buttocks implants are exactly what one might imagine—**implants that**

YOU'RE GOING ABROAD FOR...WHAT!?

shape and/or raise the buttocks area. People interested in buttocks implants should be aware of some recovery issues in addition to those expected normally. Someone who has had a butt implant will be unable to sit for at least ten days and will not be allowed to sleep on his or her back for at least a month. Prices vary, though the usual "overseas discount" of 40 to 75 percent seems to apply. Butt implants in Brazil can cost $2,500 to $3,500; I have seen costs in the United States range from $5,000 to $10,000.

Some surgeons will also do a procedure that involves injecting a patient's own fat, obtained by liposuction, into the buttocks area. This can cost $500 to $1,000 abroad, in addition to the cost of the liposuction. Results can be mixed, as some patients absorb some of the fat back into their bodies.

Butt implants have increased in popularity in recent years, as have a host of other more esoteric procedures such as refashioning the labia.

OTHER COSMETIC PROCEDURES

Hair Implants
Hair implants involve the transplantation of **thousands of tiny patches of hair-bearing scalp tissue to the balding areas of the head**. Results vary from patient to patient and are by no means guaranteed. Though Costa Rica's Dr. Cohen mentioned that he does not see as many hair transplant patients as he once did because transplantation has become less expensive in the United States, research indicates that there is still a substantial "overseas discount" of 25 to 50 percent.

Hair transplant prices are generally based on the number of hair/skin grafts done. U.S. prices range upwards from about $3,000, depending on the extent of the work.

Ear Pinning (Otoplasty)
Prior to research, I'd had no idea that fixing protruding ears was a popular cosmetic procedure. Otoplasty is the general term for **cosmetically**

enhancing the appearance of the ears. Roughly 25,000 U.S. residents underwent some sort of cosmetic surgery of the ear in 2004, according to ASPS statistics. Prices in the United States range from $2,500 to $4,000; prices abroad range from $800 to $1,500.

Weight-Loss Surgery (Bariatric Surgery)

Bariatric surgery that is designed to cause significant weight loss is increasingly popular in the United States. The surgery **alters the digestive process, either restricting the amount of food the stomach can hold or causing food not to be absorbed.** There are several different procedures and techniques with more continuing to evolve. The intestinal bypass was the first and is still the most common in the United States.

There are eight recognized types of bariatric surgery including laproscopic bariatric surgery, bariatric bypass surgery, and vertical banded gastroplasty (VBG).

Bariatric surgery is considered a drastic lifesaving solution for a major health problem. In this instance, it is covered by some medical insurance plans and prospective patients in the United States who have health insurance are generally well-advised to explore the option with their insurer. However, many patients do go abroad to afford the surgery. For those interested in bariatric surgery and wondering where to start, I recommend without qualification the ObesityHelp Web site **(www.obesityhelp.com)**, an online support group that boasts more than 200,000 members.

> Bariatric surgery is considered a drastic lifesaving solution for a major health problem.

Dental Procedures and Appliances

My personal experience with going abroad for costmetic surgery is limited to dental work. It is ironic, perhaps, I did far less research prior to going to Costa Rica for full-mouth reconstruction than I now recommend that others do before making a decision. Readers interested in the extensive details of my own experience should visit my Web site *Beauty from Afar*

(www.beautyfromafar.com).
Since having my work done in
2004, I have recommended at
least dozens of patients to Drs.
Cordero and Rubinstein at Prisma
Dental in Costa Rica. Invariably,

Dental surgery patients
going abroad generally
do not require
extended convalescence.

however, I point out that there are other excellent dentists in Costa Rica
and around the world, and I urge prospective dental patients to thoroughly
explore their options at home and abroad before making a decision.

Dental insurance in the United States rarely covers the full cost of
extensive cosmetic work. There is certainly little reason to go abroad for
routine dental work. However, when the prospective out-of-pocket
expense for wanted or needed dental work climbs into the thousands of
dollars, going overseas can become the pragmatic option.

Generally, dental patients do not require extended convalescence
abroad, or significant immediate after-care and support, as do medical
surgery patients. Costs range widely based on various dental procedures,
but my general statement that patients can expect to save from 40 to 75
percent on medical services abroad holds true for dental work. Many
cosmetic surgery patients abroad opt to get at least minor cosmetic
dental work, such as teeth whitening, done on the same trip.

WHAT ELSE IS OUT THERE?
(Non-Cosmetic Procedures)

Except for perhaps the very cutting-edge care techniques, for which the
United States maintains a still-visible edge on the rest of the world, most
surgical procedures are available elsewhere from qualified and reputable
doctors, in state-of-the art facilities, and at prices sharply below those in
the United States. The primary examples, for now, are the private, international hospitals of the Far East, most notably but not exclusively those
in **Thailand**, **India**, and **Malaysia**.

International private hospitals advertise a variety of procedures and
services, including but not limited to:

- Cardiology and cardiothoracic (open heart) surgery
- Joint replacements
- Orthopedic surgery
- Full-service gastroenterology procedures
- Eye surgery and other ophthalmology procedures
- Organ transplants
- Urology and prostate procedures

They claim to be world-class, which United States residents can take to mean equivalent to or better than what they may have access to at home. There is strong evidence that the international

> There is strong evidence that the international hospitals are as good as U.S. hospitals.

hospitals are, in fact, that good. They represent an option that the uninsured and underinsured in the United States should not ignore, if facing unaffordable and unavoidable medical expenses.

AS GOOD—OR EVEN BETTER

The prestigious International Society of Minimally Invasive Cardiothoracic Surgery (ISMICS) is an organization dominated by United States and European doctors, so it is no surprise that when Naresh Trehan, M.D., of India, was elected president in 2005, it made big news. In an interview with the *India Post* he made the following points:

- Having lived in the United State for 20 years, "I know, to get equal recognition, we [foreign doctors] have to be 150 percent better than our counterparts in America."
- "There is huge inward flow [of patients to India] from the rest of the world."
- "I'm building 'MediCity,' which will be like the Johns Hopkins or the Mayo Clinic of the East."

- "I am not in favor of advertising, but the information should be out to people that it is possible to access treatment [and get] good outcomes and affordable costs in India; and that the experience can be very positive if one chooses the right place."

Can anyone really doubt that quality medical care is available globally? In the United States and elsewhere, however, it is increasingly the responsibility of the patient to evaluate medical options and make choices. Fortunately, the research tools are widely available, and people can learn to master them.

CHAPTER 5

Research, Research, Research

Before I wrote a word of this book, I:

- Read or at least skimmed—and saved—more than 6,000 posts about medical tourism and cosmetic surgery in Internet forums. I have no idea how many I read and did *not* save.
- Accumulated more than 200 Internet bookmarks—and this is despite pruning my files regularly to try to only keep the ones I thought I absolutely needed.
- Read or at least glanced through more than 1,500 news stories and press releases about medical tourism and cosmetic surgery. I read seven or eight books, only three of which I had to buy. I found the others in the library.

My e-mail folders for book material alone number more than 40, on two separate Internet accounts. Mercifully, I have unlimited long-distance at a flat rate in North America and very inexpensive overseas rates with an Internet phone service. The time I spent on the phone with surgeons and patients and other sources was extensive, but the cost was nearly inconsequential.

I say this not to boast, but to explain that doing the research for this book did not work out at all the way I had originally hoped. It was a grind, a day-in and day-out sifting and weighing of information that went on for a year. I had wanted to travel from country to country—around the world, in fact. In between plane flights, I had wanted to live in strange and new places—perhaps, on-and-off, for months. Everyone I e-mailed, everyone I talked to on the phone, I wanted to meet in person; and I still do.

Maybe someday. It was as unaffordable for me in 2005 as the dental work I needed was in 2003. I did go to some places. In the end, I realized, more traveling would not have made for a better or more useful book, though it would have been more fun for me and better for me and my sources to meet in person. But I might have skimped on the basic research. A reader might enjoy my around-the-world tour but find it the superficial account of a jet-setter. If you are going to consider the option of going abroad for medical care or cosmetic surgery or dental work, you probably won't tour facilities in person around the globe, either. You'll sit at home and research and read, as I did. Then you'll either plan and go, or you won't.

A lot of people are very good, even great, at doing research on the Internet. They may skim through this chapter, as skilled Internet researchers, familiar with the tricks and tips I am about to unveil. But I know from years of experience working for Internet companies that most people are less than expert in their use of computers and the Internet, even to the point of feeling helpless. But you, or a friend willing to help you, will need at least rudimentary computer skills—typing, mouse clicking, Web browsing—to get what you need from this chapter.

THE BARE MINIMUM—GENERAL RESOURCES

Recommending Web sites in a book is somewhat perilous. Books are immutable. Web sites come and go, change, move, break; they can go stale; they can even be stolen. However, there are a few—just a few—in which I have a high degree of confidence, enough to recommend them in print and discuss. They are enough to get anyone well-started who is interested in traveling abroad for cosmetic surgery or any other kind of medical care.

It is certainly possible, using the following dozen or so sites to:
- Consider the cosmetic procedures in which you have an interest.
- Decide whether traveling overseas for surgery is an option you want to consider.
- Evaluate options as to which country to go to, which surgeon to consult, and where to stay.

You'd still have a whole lot of e-mails, phone calls, planning, and worrying ahead of you, but between this book and the Web sites provided, you should be able to glean enough to make informed decisions. You might make a few new virtual friends, as well.

In most countries—the United States included—any licensed medical doctor can legally perform many cosmetic procedures and surgeries. Checking credentials and references is critical, whether your prospective surgeon is in the United States or abroad. When asked about a "south-of-the-border" cosmetic surgery disaster story, one Mexican surgeon simply told me: "There are charlatans everywhere. The United States has them. We have them. People have to be careful."

I have known people to make a decision to travel abroad for cosmetic surgery and/or dental care on as little as the advice of one good friend. I've known others who agonized over the decision for months, researching perhaps as much as I did to write this book before making up their minds. Most people fall somewhere in between.

The big Internet search sites are a paramount tool, of course. I prefer **Google (www.google.com)**, more out of habit than any firm conviction that it is the best, and will cite examples of using Google for searching and other services. I have no relationship of any sort with Google that compels me to mention it or cite its usefulness; I am simply used to working with it. However, if you are more comfortable with other search engines, or prefer using multiple search engines, I can not say that you will have any less success. Use what works for you. I will have occasion to mention **Yahoo (www.yahoo.com)** and **MSN (www.msn.com)** as well.

You will be able to find updated links and information at the support site for this book, **www.beautyfromafar.com.**

GENERAL SITES

There are many **U.S. government sites** that are overwhelmingly useful for reference to anyone researching medical care online. Two are **National Institutes of Health (www.nih.gov)** and its associated site for the **National Library of Medicine (www.nlm.nih.gov)**. A third site worth adding to your favorites is **Healthfinder (www.healthfinder.gov)**. These sites are well-organized, well-maintained, searchable, and, all in all, good starting points for researching health and medical issues.

There are dozens, even hundreds, of member societies, associations, and organizations for medical professionals in the United States alone that provide useful information for consumers and patients as well. There are also such sites in many other countries—but most are not in English. If you read and speak Spanish, you have an edge. Other languages may help as well, particularly Portuguese, if you are interested in Brazil.

However, unless otherwise noted, I will be referring to sites that have English-language versions available. While Google and many other sites have translation tools, they are far from perfect. I have, however, found it to be very useful for at least getting the gist of non-English-language sites.

COSMETIC SURGERY SITES

Whether you are considering going abroad for cosmetic surgery or not, the Web sites of the main professional associations for board-certified plastic and cosmetic surgeons in the United States are first-rate resources for news and researching procedures.

American Society of Plastic Surgeons

www.plasticsurgery.org

The American Society of Plastic Surgeons (ASPS) is the largest plastic surgery specialty organization in the world. Founded in 1931, the society comprises board-certified plastic surgeons who perform cosmetic and reconstructive surgery.

American Society for Aesthetic Plastic Surgery

www.surgery.org

The 2,200-member **American Society for Aesthetic Plastic Surgery (ASAPS)** is devoted entirely to the advancement of cosmetic surgery. ASAPS is recognized throughout the world as the authoritative source for cosmetic surgery education. U.S. members are certified by the American Board of Plastic Surgery. Canadian members are certified in plastic surgery by the Royal College of Physicians and Surgeons of Canada.

American Academy of Facial Plastic and Reconstructive Surgery

www.aafprs.org

The **American Academy of Facial Plastic and Reconstructive Surgery (AAFPRS)** represents 2,800 facial plastic and reconstructive surgeons throughout the world. The majority of AAFPRS members are certified by the American Board of Otolaryngology, which includes passing an exam in facial plastic and reconstructive procedures. Other AAFPRS members are surgeons certified in ophthalmology, plastic surgery, and dermatology.

American Academy of Cosmetic Surgery

www.cosmeticsurgery.org

The **American Academy of Cosmetic Surgery (AACS)** is a professional medical society whose members are dedicated to patient safety and physician education in cosmetic surgery. Most members of the AACS are dermatologic surgeons, facial plastic surgeons, head and neck surgeons, general surgeons, oral and maxillofacial surgeons, plastic surgeons, or ocular plastic surgeons—all of whom may specialize in cosmetic surgery.

Regardless of the concerns and misgivings that many surgeons in the United States express about patients traveling abroad for surgery, the AACS has partnered with Dubai Healthcare City in the United Arab Emirates to build the American Academy of Cosmetic Surgery Hospital. The hospital will "include a cosmetic surgery hospital and academic facilities and bring world-class institutions and learning events to Dubai Healthcare City," according to the AACS Web site. Construction began in mid-2005, the hospital was scheduled to be completed in mid-2006. For more information, browse to **www.dhcc.ae.**

The International Society of Aesthetic Plastic Surgery

www.isaps.org

The International Society of Aesthetic Plastic Surgery (ISAPS) is the international society representing plastic surgeons that specialize in aesthetic plastic surgery and the official aesthetic plastic surgery chapter of the **International Confederation of Plastic, Reconstructive, and Aesthetic Plastic Surgery (IPRAS) (www.ipras.org)**.

As of January 2006, ISAPS listed 1,316 total dues-paying member surgeons from 67 countries. Membership is by invitation only; contact information for member surgeons is available on the site, including e-mail addresses for many and Web sites for some. The United States has more members than any other country, with 188. Brazil has 165; Mexico, 133.

ISAPS members compose a very small percentage of the total number of surgeons worldwide who are board-certified by national organizations with standards comparable to those in the United States. It is an elite group of sorts, but keep in mind that while some of the best cosmetic surgeons in the world are members, many more of the best are not members.

OTHER SITES

There are many international societies or associations of board-certified cosmetic and plastic surgeons that have Web sites, some with English-language versions. They can include very good general information to help in your research. One of the best is the **Mexican Association of Plastic, Aesthetic and Reconstructive Surgery (AMCPER)** site **(www.plasticsurgery.org.mx)**. In Mexico, board-certification signifies a surgeon has had at least 6 years of surgical training, 3 of them in plastic surgery, after graduating from medical school, and has passed certification exams—roughly equivalent to the certification process in the United States.

PATIENT SUPPORT SITES

For months, I wondered what was the most useful information I could put in this chapter when it came time to write it. Then it came to me. There are a number of forums on the Internet for patients to discuss cosmetic surgery, and there are many Web sites put up by patients who have been abroad for surgery. There are also a growing number of commercial Web sites that help connect prospective patients with overseas surgeons and even make all the arrangements for a surgery trip. I'll talk about some of them as we go along, but these are the important, can't-do-without-them Web sites. As it turns out, the best support site for patients who are looking into the option of going overseas for cosmetic surgery evolved before my eyes.

Plastic Surgery Journeys

www.plasticsurgeryjourneys.com or **www.psjourneys.com**

PlasticSurgeryJourneys.com (PSJ), which used to be strictly a message group, has truly lived up to its promise of working toward being **the best international plastic surgery resource and support group on the Web**. Registration is required but membership is free as long as you post a message at least every 2 weeks. A premium membership, for those who don't want to be held to the posting requirement or who simply want to support the site, is around $35 a year.

What sets PSJ apart is both the commitment of its founders and the quality and passion of its membership. The site has evolved rapidly, thanks to both. The forums are a trove of information compiled by a researching and questing army of patients and interested potential patients. If you want to read about the experiences that others have had in traveling abroad for cosmetic surgery, talk about choosing a surgeon, get advice in any aspect of planning your trip, or just crave a little company and moral support, PSJ is where you want to be looking.

I drop in almost daily to see what's new; as I type this, I notice that 55 people have answered the survey on "How much money would you say you have saved by having plastic surgery done outside the United States?" More than two-thirds of the respondents have chosen answers indicating an amount greater than $5,000.

ObesityHelp

www.obesityhelp.com

This site is a terrific resource for those considering weight-loss surgery. However, it is also a great site for anyone considering cosmetic surgery abroad. There is a voluminous message board for plastic-surgery patients, reviews of international surgeons, and a membership directory. Even if you are not obese, it's well worth a look-through if you are interested in cosmetic surgery—particularly on the body rather than the face.

MEDICAL AND TRAVEL SERVICES

There is an entire industry growing up around the notion that medical tourism is "the next big thing," or at least one of the next big things. Hospitals and surgeons in developing countries are not the only entities interested. Companies are springing up that will handle most of the details for prospective patients. One such company is the U.S.-based firm **MedRetreat (www.medretreat.com)**, which was launched in the spring of 2005 and offers a full array of medical services in a number of countries. Individuals are starting businesses as medical tourist guides and booking agents for surgeons, and resorts and destinations are seeking to add medical services to their array of lures.

None of these patient-services companies has emerged as a leader yet, but I will continue to track companies and their services on my Web site: **www.beautyfromafar.com.**

GENERAL TOURISM

There are a seemingly infinite number of Web sites devoted to international tourism and travel, and they're easy to find. However, I have a personal favorite that is appropriate as the final "must visit" site: **Virtual Tourist (VT) (www.virtualtourist.com)**. VT boasts more than 600,000 members from more than 220 countries and territories. Wherever you might want to go, whatever your questions might be, you can find someone at VT who has "been there, done that." Free registration is not required but is necessary to participate in some areas of the site.

In addition, I advise spending some time looking around at **travel.state.gov**, the U.S. State Department's official site for international travel. There you will find information on all paperwork requirements for foreign travel; tips and warnings for traveling abroad, by country; and advice on health, safety, and emergency services.

NUMBER ONE PRIORITY: GOOD RESEARCH

The sites noted in this chapter are sufficient for anyone to begin and finalize a decision to travel abroad for cosmetic surgery. Consider them a baseline and prime points of entry. The next level—a step beyond my arbitrary but informed site recommendations—is the rest of the Internet. You'll be searching it, of course. Below are my best tips, customized for searching for information about medical tourism and cosmetic surgery in different countries. Your results will not be exactly the same, of course—search returns can change almost minute-to-minute, and the numbers below are an example, a snapshot in time.

Using Search Engines

Whatever search engine you use—remember, I'm using Google—most of the following tips and observations can be generalized.

Using Quotation Marks

This is one of the most useful search limiters available, and even people who are well aware of it rarely use it to full advantage. When searching for an exact phrase or sequence of words, enclose the phrase or sequence in quotes when searching. Example:

Search for	Total results
medical tourism	21,400,000
"medical tourism"	326,000

Using Multiple Terms

Be as specific as you can get—using more terms is better. And continue to set off exact phrases and sequences in quotes. Example:

Search for	Total results
medical tourism cosmetic surgery	2,470,000
"medical tourism" "cosmetic surgery"	14,900

Using Country Names

Unless you specify the name of another country in your search, your results will be dominated by United States sites. If you're looking for information about cosmetic surgery overseas, it may save you a lot of time and frustration to look country by country, specifying those that interest you. Example:

RESEARCH, RESEARCH, RESEARCH

Search for	Total results
"cosmetic surgery"	9,650,000
"cosmetic surgery" "Costa Rica"	492,000

Using Synonyms and Similar Phrases

Try different words and different word orders. Use "aesthetic" or "plastic" instead of or in addition to "cosmetic." Use both "procedure" and "surgery." Try "liposuction," then try "lipo." You'll get a variety of results and different returns in your first few search result pages. Example:

Search for	Total results
"cosmetic surgery" "Costa Rica"	492,000
"cosmetic surgery" "Costa Rica" "aesthetic"	23,700

Using Key Phrases and Words You Might Expect to Find

Think about the kind of page you are hoping to find. If you were writing the content for that page, consider what words and phrases you might use. Example:

Search for	Total results
"cosmetic surgery" "Costa Rica"	492,000
"cosmetic surgery" "Costa Rica" "inexpensive" "less than in the U.S."	6

Remember that returning fewer results is not always better. In the above example, you do get six interesting links but none of them are for doctors or medical facilities. However, it's something to play around with, something to think about, something with which you can be creative. I was amused at the results I got when adding phrases such as "best in the world" or "world's best." The results were not terribly useful, but it was interesting to see who might make such claims on a Web page.

Get Even More Specific

Once you have the names of some specific doctors or surgeons, search using their full names as well, even if you have found Web sites for their practices. Often, or at least sometimes, you'll be able to find additional information, like patient reviews of their own experiences or if the doctors are associated with any professional organizations. Example:

Search for	Total results
face-lift Mexico	498,000
face-lift Mexico "Jaime Caloca"	517

Using Country Codes and Advanced Search

Everyone has heard of "dot coms." The majority of the addresses of Internet Web sites end in .com. Dot com addresses will generally dominate your search results, with other domain suffixes (.org, .net, .edu, .gov, individual country suffixes) getting lost in the crowd.

A complete list of country codes can be found by searching "Internet country code." Here are the codes for the nations that are among the most common medical-tourism destinations:

Argentina	.ar	**India**	.in
Brazil	.br	**Malaysia**	.my
Colombia	.co	**Mexico**	.mx
Costa Rica	.cr	**South Africa**	.za
Czech Republic	.cz	**Spain**	.es
Dominican Republic	.do	**Thailand**	.th
Hungary	.hu	**United States**	.us

Using Google's Advanced Search (linked from Google's main page), you can search just these lesser-known and lesser-used domain suffixes to your advantage. Limit your search to just .org sites, and you will see many more associations and nonprofit organizations. Limit your search to .edu sites, and you will find more academic research. By limiting your search to just Web sites with a particular country code suffix, you will see many Web sites that would otherwise likely be buried deeply within your search results. Some of them will certainly not be in English—but once you have found them, you can filter and see only the ones that are, if you so choose.

There are two ways to limit your search by domain. One is by using the Google Advanced Search page. There are two options associated with using the "domain" filter. You can first choose whether you want to get results *only* having a particular domain suffix versus results from which you *exclude* a domain suffix; and, second, you choose a domain suffix. For this second part, type in only a period followed by the suffix or country code. For example: .org, .edu, .mx, .br.

Let's say, for example, searching for "plastic surgery" and limiting the search only to the country code for Hungary (.hu) yields about 700 results, some of them probably of interest to anyone contemplating plastic surgery in that country. Searching the more traditional way for "plastic surgery" "Hungary" without the country code limiter gets 36,600 results, with the list top-heavy with dot com sites. Both searches may be useful.

The second way to limit your search by domain is to use the regular Google search page but type: "search term" site domain suffix or country ᴑde. So one would type "plastic surgery" site:.hu into the main Google search box to get the same result as one would get using the Google Advanced Search page in the previous example. Typing "medical tourism" site:.org or "medical tourism" site:.edu brings up a different array of perspectives on the subject of medical tourism than does a more general search. Try it!

Google News Alerts

There are a variety of services on the Internet that will track news events related to your individual interests. Google searches more than 4,500 news sources and sends me daily e-mail links to reports that contain my search criteria. To add your own criteria for this service, go to the **Google news page (news.google.com)** and click on "news alerts." My own news alerts are for:

> **"medical tourism"**
> **"health tourism"**
> **"plastic surgery"**
> **"cosmetic surgery"**
> **"aesthetic surgery"**

On any given day, I might receive up to five news alerts with links to stories containing these search phrases. There is overlap, of course; and many of the links that are sent to me are of no particular use or interest. But, overall, using news alerts is a magnificent and efficient way to become generally informed about a given topic over time.

You, of course, can use less-general search criteria and make your own alerts more specific in exactly the same way as you would with a regular one-time search of the Internet or of a news site.

Google Ads

When you search, pay some attention to the ads placed on the results page. I'm not talking about pop-up ads, but the text ads that are generated when you type in particular words or phrases and are included along with your search results on the right-hand side. This is all part of the money-making machine of search-engine companies. People and companies pay to have their text ads appear—and, sometimes, it is these ads that will deliver the information for which you're looking.

For example, during my research, I ran across a medical tourism search site, **Firefly International (www.fireflymed.com)**, in the ads. Firefly, among other things, says it is "an online Web portal for individuals seeking elective, cosmetic, or surgical procedures not covered by their personal health-care insurance." Interested? Sure I am. Are they any good, will they be around 6 months or a year from now? Maybe, maybe not. But they are apparently one of the many start-up companies interested in profiting from medical tourism by providing services to prospective patients. The point is, I found them through their ad, not through direct search results.

Using Translation Tools

Google provides a language-translation link that may occasionally be of use for reading or interpreting content you find on the Web. Computer translations are imperfect and incomplete, at times even wildly and hilariously so. Also, even though translation tools can attempt to translate entire Web pages, some pages are designed in such a way that thwart your attempt at translating them. Despite this, translation services can be occasionally useful for phrases and figuring out the navigation of sites in foreign languages.

For example, having a handy translation tool helped me decipher the navigation of the Portuguese-language Web site of the Brazilian Society of Plastic Surgeons at least to the point where I could access and use the searchable member directory.

Bookmarking and/or Saving Favorites

Saved Web pages are called bookmarks by most Internet browsing tools, though Microsoft Internet Explorer, the most commonly used browser, calls them Favorites. Whatever you use, you will want to save the locations of sites to which you may want to refer again. Look in the top menu bar of your browser and click on "Bookmarks" or "Favorites." Use the pull-down menus for adding, saving, filing, and organizing the sites you want to keep.

You will also want to bookmark an online currency converter. Yahoo has a good one that is easy to use, but there are many. Prices for procedures are not always converted for you.

Finding and Using Groups

Access to many special-interest groups exists just beyond the reach of routine Web searching. The major Internet services—**AOL**, **MSN**, and **Yahoo**, for starters—give individuals the ability to start groups that can develop into significant social and informational entities. They can also stagnate, disappear, or be nothing more than conduits for junk e-mail. As of this writing, I've found most of the useful groups to be on Yahoo. I found little of interest on MSN and nothing on AOL, but remember that special interest and support groups can spring up out of nowhere and take on a life of their own. Search for "cosmetic surgery" and/or other relevant terms at **groups.yahoo.com** or **groups.msn.com**.

You will have to register for a free account with Yahoo or MSN, respectively, to join or participate in groups.

Of particular note on Yahoo are groups for Costa Rica and Brazil that are run by patients who have had surgery in one of those countries, by medical tourism companies, and even by individual surgeons. There are similar groups for other countries that are (so far) not as active. In September 2005, for example, I belonged to approximately 20 different Yahoo groups devoted to cosmetic surgery or medical tourism in some way. Most of them seem inactive but a few of them have significant memberships, interesting discussions, and extensive file and photo sections. One such group that has been in existence for a number of years is **Rosenstock_Lieberman_Clinic_ Costa_Rica_Plastic_Surgery.** Though the group is specifically a support site for one prominent Costa Rican cosmetic surgery practice, the Rosenstock-Lieberman Center for Cosmetic Plastic Surgery, there are more than 1,000 members and a wealth of general resources are available.

Some people are reluctant to join forums or groups online, perhaps out of shyness or embarrassment at being new, or out of concern for anonymity and privacy. To them I can only say to work past your worries. Groups and forums can be fractious, confusing, and sometimes an utter waste of time to keep up with, yes; but there is no better resource for making up your mind about whether to go overseas for surgery or medical care than personal testimony. The previously mentioned patient support Web sites or online groups can get you in touch with people whose stories and lessons could fill volumes, but personal stories are already available to you online.

Using E-mail (Communicating with Surgeons)

You're going to be using e-mail quite a bit in communicating with prospective surgeons and/or staff. Here are a few tips on how to do it and what to expect:

1. **Surgeons and doctors who have experience in serving patients from abroad are quite accustomed to dealing with e-mail inquiries.** Your initial inquiry can be a general request for information about the surgeon's credentials, rough prices for procedures, and references. The surgeon, his or her staff, or a representative will likely respond with something that reads like a form letter. This is a good sign, actually—it means they're used to this, and the letter should answer most of your preliminary questions. The form letter will also tell you what the surgeon requires of you in order to ascertain if you are a suitable patient, to determine a treatment or surgery plan, and an estimate of costs. Generally, this will involve you sending digital photographs to the surgeon and some medical history. If you are looking into dental work, it will help the overseas dentist tremendously to see recent x-rays. The surgeon or doctor will let you know what he or she needs; you can volunteer anything additional that you think may help.

2. **Don't expect perfect English.** I have learned not to expect doctors and surgeons or staff in foreign countries to have perfect command

of written English. For that matter, I have learned not to expect that in the United States, either. What is important is to ask and follow up on anything that is not clear. Use simple and direct language. English is tricky enough for those of us who speak and write nothing else daily. Even surgeons who speak English fluently as a second or third language will stumble on uncommon words or slang in speech or in writing. They want to understand you and will ask if they are uncertain. For your part, be vigilant about being satisfied with the answers that you get.

3. **Do not expect immediate responses via e-mail**, though you may get some. Allow someone several days before following up (or giving up). People do get exceptionally busy, or go away for a few days.

4. **You should be able, at some point, to talk to your surgeon on the telephone.** Schedule this appointment via e-mail. You should not count on him or her being available if you just call cold. Presumably, just like doctors in the United States, they spend most of their time treating and operating on patients. Stick primarily with e-mail, which also leaves you with a record of what you have been told.

5. **It is not unreasonable to ask a surgeon for references from other patients whom you can contact directly.** They expect this. Something is wrong if they can not provide them. Patients who have had good experiences in traveling abroad for cosmetic surgery are generally happy to talk or write about it.

6. **Generally, a surgeon who is used to an international clientele will have recommendations on local accommodations.** Feel free to ask for his or her suggestions on travel arrangements as well.

7. **Follow your instincts.** If you are unable to build a rapport with a surgeon and/or his or her staff, you can't get your questions answered to your satisfaction, have difficulty getting references, or you can not

verify a surgeon's credentials—anything that makes you feel uncomfortable—you should consider consulting a different surgeon.

8. **Keep copies of all correspondence.** Take them with you on your trip.

Taking and Sending Photos

For some reason, this request flummoxes some people. But if you want to have cosmetic surgery abroad, you are going to need some high-quality and possibly very unflattering or embarrassing digital photos of yourself. If you are interested only in facial work, perhaps it is not so bad, but the surgeon will still want to see close-ups from a number of angles and a description of what you want done to improve your appearance. If you are interested in various cosmetic procedures on your body, a surgeon will need to see nude photos from various angles.

You may have to resize the photos to suit your surgeon. Some e-mail services limit the size of attachments. Consult with your surgeon's office before sending photos. Although some people may have reservations about sending photos, especially nude photos, via the Internet, it is the fastest, most convenient way to send them, and it is probably more reliable than international mail.

CHAPTER 6

There and Back Again

I was nearly home from my last trip to Costa Rica, riding a shuttle bus late at night from Bradley International Airport in Windsor Locks, Connecticut, to where my ancient Subaru had been parked for a week, some five miles away. There was one other guy on the bus.

"Where you coming from?" I asked.

"Florida. Miami. We have a place down there. Did a little fishing," he said. "You?"

"Costa Rica. Had some dental work done," I replied, admiring our brevity.

"Dental work. Really." He said it more by way of a pause than in disbelief. Finally, he added, "So did you see one of those voodoo doctors?" I blanched, hearing it for that moment as a deadly insult, just as my Costa Rican friends might have. But I could tell the guy wasn't trying to be mean. He just didn't know, and was making a joke; he was waiting for an answer. So I gave him the short version—that health care in Costa Rica is first rate, and cheap, besides. I really couldn't tell if it made much of an impression. I didn't think to expand and tell him how much I liked San José or about the wonderful restaurants and nightlife, or the shopping. Maybe I should have mentioned the beautiful women. But it was late, and the bus ride was short.

***

Americans residing in the United States have something of a reputation internationally for not having seen much of the world that is beyond their own borders. That only about 18 percent of the United States population have passports is considered by some, at home and abroad, as evidence of poor world citizenship and bad national character. This is something of a bum rap. It is easy to take the other side of the argument, and point out that while the number of U.S. citizens who have passports does sound pretty low, those who have them use them quite a bit. More than 27 million

Americans (about 9 percent of the population) went abroad in 2004 for one reason or another, according to the U.S. Department of Commerce. That's approximately the entire population of New York and New Jersey combined, which makes it sound like a lot; and it's 8 million less than the population of California, which somehow makes it sound like not quite so many. It all depends on how you want to look at it.

Still, it is a fact that the vast majority of U.S. citizens rarely go overseas, and that it is mostly the same people who do go year in and year out. Not surprisingly, people who do travel internationally tend to have higher incomes than most, in the six-figure neighborhood on average. Presumably, with the income comes decent medical insurance, and fewer qualms about paying U.S. prices for elective procedures. Those most likely to be looking for inexpensive health care or cosmetic surgery abroad, by reason of limited finances, are also less likely to be experienced international travelers.

Even for those who are used to planning extended trips abroad for vacation or for business, this is different. This trip abroad must be constructed around medical necessities, physical incapacity, and recovery.

MISCONCEPTIONS

What do you think when you think of Thailand, India, or Malaysia? Of Mexico, or Costa Rica and any other Central American country? Of Brazil, or South America? Of Eastern Europe, or South Africa?

Odds are, you don't know much, which will tend to make you at least a little suspicious and fearful. You have heard these countries referred to as "third world" or "underdeveloped." So you think poverty, crime, poor transportation, a lack of amenities—something both less than and other than what you are used to at home.

And you can find all of those things, if you are looking for them. You may well see poverty on the way from the airport to wherever you are staying, or in neighborhoods through which you are driven. You will be warned of street crime and robberies. The roads may be in disrepair. (We are somewhat used to this in Connecticut and New York, anyway; I thought the roads in Costa Rica were fine, but the locals complained bitterly of the potholes.) The amenities will be different; the foods somewhat different; the customs different. However, you can generally choose the degree to which you want to be insulated. Your doctor or surgeon will insist on it, at least to an extent. In truth, there are no indignities to be endured in these places that you would not find in Miami, New York, Dallas, Chicago, or Los Angeles. Language is the biggest difficulty for many, but everywhere you go you will find people who speak English. You will be told that you can drink the water, but it is easy to find it in bottles if you prefer. Choose your surgeons or doctors well, consult with them and other medical tourists on accommodations, and your biggest problems will be coping with the discomfort or pain of convalescence after surgery, and with the associated boredom.

I was nervous about going to Costa Rica for the first time, even though I have spent time in Europe and in Africa; you'd think I would have known better. Though I was only having dental work, I

> You can choose the degree to which you will be insulated. Your doctor will insist on it.

stayed initially for a few days at a recovery retreat for surgical patients. I was met at the airport, shuttled to and from my dental appointments, and I relaxed in relatively inexpensive luxury with mostly fellow North Americans. The food was excellent. Roughly $100 a day covered all my expenses. After three days, two of them spent mostly in a dentist's chair, I was confident enough of Costa Rica to want to see more, and moved to a hotel downtown. I walked 20 minutes or took a cab to the dentists' office. I wandered the city by day, but was cautious at night. I had a splendid time for a week, fitting in several inexpensive tours of coffee-growing country, a volcano, a rain forest, and of San José itself. My biggest inconvenience was not speaking or understanding Spanish, but that never caused any more than temporary frustration or embarrassment. One can expect similar circumstances in any metropolitan area sophisticated and pragmatic enough to be courting North American tourists and their dollars.

CHOOSING A COUNTRY

Most people who travel abroad for cosmetic surgery, dental work, or other medical care will tell you that their journey began when their research did. Even without leaving home, they had to imagine themselves abroad, create a picture in their minds of a successful trip. For some, this takes weeks. Others are taking the trip in their heads for months.

If you have personal ties to a particular country that is also a prime medical tourist destination, your choice is probably simple. Pick that country, then look for a doctor or surgeon. If you have reason to prefer a particular surgeon, you're going to go to wherever he or she practices. But if you're starting from scratch, I'd advise picking a country first, or at least a region, based on personal preferences. It need not have anything to do with medical care. There are, in fact, good doctors and surgeons almost everywhere. Picking a country first will help narrow your search. You can change your mind later.

I chose Costa Rica over Thailand for dental work not because I thought the dentists were better, but mostly because it is closer to home for me. Proximity counted; I'd much rather spend four hours on airplanes than 16 to get to my destination. The airfare is far less expensive, which offset, to some extent, the price advantage that Thailand seemed to have. I also considered Mexico but, coming from Connecticut, there seemed no additional convenience to going there; and there was far more information available on the Internet about Costa Rican dentists than there was about Mexican dentists.

In general, I have found that the farther away from the United States you go for medical services, the lower the price will be. Thailand, India, and Malaysia are somewhat less expensive than Central and South America. There are exceptions, of course. South Africa is farther away and is not that much less expensive (though it has its own allure for many, myself included). But the lower prices in Asia are offset at least in part by higher travel costs. There is a tradeoff to factor in. If you live in the deep Southwest United States, Mexico may be your natural choice for medical tourism just because you can drive there.

I know one woman who wants to go to Brazil for her tummy tuck. She is aware of the country's outstanding reputation for cosmetic surgery, but that is not why she is choosing Brazil over other destinations. She is choosing Brazil because she has always wanted to go there. Even though she will spend much of her time in Rio de Janeiro or São Paulo recovering from surgery, and not at the beach or dancing the nights away, Brazil is where she wants to go.

> The farther away you get from the United States, the cheaper it will be.

You're not going anywhere, in your head, until you pick a place. That's where your journey begins.

MEDICAL TOURISM COMPANIES

If you want professional help planning your journey, it is available. There are a small but growing number of companies that cater specifically to the needs of medical tourists. One such company is **MedRetreat (www.medretreat.com)**, which I mentioned in the previous chapter. I use it as a model because I have met the principals and am comfortable that they have done their homework and are committed to customer and patient services. But there are others, many, I'm sure, equally as fine.

These companies are set up to walk you through the entire experience. Besides helping you choose and communicate with a foreign doctor or surgeon, they provide full travel services, an English-speaking guide in your destination country, and safety and accountability of financial transactions with the foreign doctor, surgeon, and/or medical facility.

Medical tourism companies are in business to make money, of course, so using one will be more expensive than going it alone. But the help will be well worth the extra cost to some travelers. In your research, you will run across everything from full-service medical tourism companies to individuals who arrange patient services for a single surgeon. In all cases, check references and make sure you know all of the costs and benefits up front. In medical tourism, bad help is far worse than no help.

TRAVELING ALONE

The first thing to know about traveling abroad alone for medical care is that people do it all the time. By "people," I mean, more pointedly, "unaccompanied women." In fact, women traveling alone for cosmetic and aesthetic surgery account for a large percentage, maybe even a majority, of medical tourists coming out of North America. Yes, some people do travel with spouses, significant others, mothers, daughters, sisters, or friends who can be along either as fellow patients or simply for companionship. Keep in mind that for at least one of you, this isn't really a vacation—it is a trip to the hospital and a period of convalescence. For this reason,

> Women traveling alone for plastic surgery probably account for a majority of the medical tourists from the United States.

experienced medical tourists express some alarm at those who desire to make the trip sort of "a family vacation," with children in tow. It can be done, of course—if you have a near perfect spouse who can manage everyone's needs, including yours. But no one recommends it. Your trip is about you, what you want, and what you need, and those who can not embrace that idea are better off left at home.

THE PASSPORT AND VISA

If you don't have a passport, make it your top priority to get one as soon as you start getting serious about going out of the country for medical care. Though it is possible to do at the last minute, it can be significantly more expensive, and the experience will probably include some inconvenience and worry, possibly to the point of panic.

Complete information about obtaining a U.S. passport for the first time, or renewing one, is available at the U.S. Department of State's travel Web site at: **www.travel.state.gov**.

Even if you are planning a trip to a country that does not require a passport for entry from the United States (such as Mexico), you should strongly consider getting one, anyway. It's a valuable and useful document to have; it's sturdier and more travel-worthy than your birth certificate and other identification. Requirements for entry into foreign countries can and do change, but a passport remains the standard travel document.

After obtaining a passport, you will need to check on any other paperwork requirements, such as visas. Again, requirements can change. Search at **www.travel.state.gov** for "foreign entry requirements." The top result, or near to it, will be a page with the list of requirements to enter any country.

MONEY

When it comes to money for medical tourism, take more than you think you'll need, and make sure you will have access to emergency funds. Check ahead of time with your surgeon and the place where you plan to stay to find out what they will accept for payment and when payment is required. Do not assume that personal checks will be acceptable. Do not even assume that traveler's checks or credit cards are acceptable. Make sure you know in advance.

There are surgeons, doctors, and facilities that will only accept cash, or that will offer discounts for payment in cash. Many medical tourists are okay with this and you can read online about the precautions people take in traveling with large sums of cash, which include sewing it within undergarments, among other measures.

> Take more money than you think you'll need.

Some medical tourism companies make a point of caring for the primary financial transactions; I consider this a significant service. If you carry more than $10,000 out of the United States, you are required by law to declare it when going through customs. Some people do and some people don't. You can find isolated examples of people who have had difficulty and delays with either choice.

I put my dental bill on credit cards and was happy to be able to do so. However, I should have alerted my credit card companies in advance that I planned to be running up significant charges overseas. To my consternation, two of my cards were initially rejected. Attempting to put thousands of dollars on them from outside the United States probably triggered every computerized fraud alarm in existence at American Express and MasterCard, and I had to spend some time on the phone from Costa Rica with each, verifying my identity and that the cards were in my physical possession.

Check in advance, also, for information about access to automated teller machines. U.S. dollars are acceptable for most transactions in many countries. It's a good idea to carry singles for tipping, but you will probably want to carry some local currency as well. Money can be exchanged in banks, but it is generally more convenient to do it where you are staying. Familiarize yourself with the exchange rate.

The worst medical tourism travel stories I have heard, besides the obvious ones about bad surgery and complications, have had to do with money—specifically, with patients who were either traveling and paying for their trips with what amounted to their life savings, or patients who had made no provisions whatsoever for unanticipated expenses. Don't put yourself in that position.

WHAT TO TAKE

I laugh aloud at even the idea of me telling a woman how to dress for a drive to the mall, let alone pack for a trip abroad. I won't even touch on clothing other than to remind you that this is more about convalescing than vacationing. If you are having cosmetic surgery on your torso, you need to take lightweight, loose-fitting clothing. If you're having a breast lift and/or breast augmentation/reduction, consult with your surgeon on what bras or support garments you may need that you can bring from home. There are a few other tips:

- If you have your own preferred pain medication, take it with you from home, as you may not be able to get the exact equivalent abroad. Check with your doctor or surgeon.

- If you have medical insurance, check before you go to determine whether it is valid when you travel abroad and, assuming it is, bring your insurance ID. Even if you are having cosmetic or other elective surgery, some treatment, including complications, may be covered by insurance.
- If you take a hair dyrer or other electrical items, throw a couple of three-way adapters in your bag. I know this isn't just a "guy thing." I carried with me what amounts to a portable office—laptop, handheld, router, battery chargers, Internet phone, etc.—and the adapters were absolutely necessary.
- If you need to stay in touch with home via phone, explore your options. You can buy international phone cards before you go, or you may be able to use your own cell phone. Check with your provider about service and rates in your destination country.
- Though you'll be surrounded by new sights and sounds, caring and interesting people, and staying in modern accommodations with amenities, you should go prepared to entertain yourself. Books. Handcrafts. Whatever it is that you like to do that's portable—bring it. You're probably not going to feel like doing much other than resting and taking it easy for at least a few days, perhaps longer, depending on what type of surgery or surgeries you have. If it matters to you, check ahead to find out what television stations are available where you're staying. Bring a portable DVD player if you have one. Even if where you're staying has a DVD player, it may not play DVDs purchased in the United States due to copyright restrictions and encryption.
- Check online for packing tips specific to the country where you're headed. People are happy to relate their own experiences.

FLYING

Well, I admit—I assume that you're flying. If you're driving to Mexico, instead, I only know enough to be nervous on your behalf. Similarly, I once got an e-mail from someone very interested in going to Costa Rica for dental work—except that he wouldn't fly, and wanted advice on getting there any other way. You can get there by ship, by car, and possibly even by bus. But I wouldn't do it, and I couldn't help him with it.

Flying is flying, but there are some applicable tips for medical tourists beyond the obligatory "shop around for the cheapest fare." First of all, check on the so-called high season (prime vacation time) for traveling to your destination country. If you're looking to save money on the flight and possibly on accommodations as well, you'll probably want to schedule your surgery and trip in a less-traveled part of the year. Some cosmetic surgeons overseas also reduce prices slightly during less-busy times of the year.

> Some cosmetic surgeons also reduce prices slightly during less busy times of the year.

It is not always possible to get direct flights to overseas destinations, but if you can, it's worth at least a little extra money, particularly for the trip home. You are not going to be at full strength—remember, you just had surgery—and you want your trip home to be as simple and stress-free as it possibly can be. Having to change planes, especially at a major hub airport, is nearly always exhausting and frustrating. Consider arranging for wheelchair service by calling the airline in advance. Even if it makes you feel a little helpless, you'll be glad afterward not to have had to walk what will seem like miles carrying or pushing luggage to get through customs and make your connecting flight.

International airports are alike the world over. You won't have any difficulty getting information and help in English.

LOCAL TRANSPORTATION

Depending on where you go, this can be either a major concern or the least of your worries. It is likely that you can arrange to be picked up at the airport and taken to wherever you are staying. Transportation to and from your medical appointments and surgery may also be a service that is handled on your behalf. Know in advance. Consult with the management at the hotel or resort where you will be staying about transportation during your visit. The safety of guests is their top priority. Make sure to take with you the addresses and phone numbers for both your doctor and for where you are staying.

ACCOMMODATIONS AND MEALS

Consult with your doctor early on regarding accommodations. Doctors who are used to having clients from abroad will have established relationships with local hotels, spas, or recovery retreats. If they don't have strong suggestions or even requirements regarding accommodations and postoperative care, you are justified in being suspicious.

Find out if you will require special meals or specific foods at any time during your stay, especially if you are having weight-loss surgery. Check ahead on the particulars and availability. Some patients do end up bringing their own protein supplements or favorite snacks, but most foods will be available locally.

RECOVERY AND AFTERCARE

Your recovery depends on following your surgeon's advice—and that includes being cleared to fly home. Inquire ahead of time regarding the average recovery time. Keep in mind, though, that not everyone heals at the same speed. Also ask what the longest recovery time could be. Allow this extra time in your schedule, since you may end up not having a choice. Remember, flights can be changed. Your health comes first.

FINALLY...OF WARNINGS

I recall a gentleman from New York who called me in the spring of 2005. He told me he was starting a medical tourism business that would cater to patients who wanted to have dental work, eye surgery, and cosmetic surgery in Colombia. I was a little skeptical.

"Going to Colombia is a tough sell in the United States," I suggested.

He knew what I meant. Say "Colombia" to the average American, and medical care is not what comes to mind, at least not until after they've finished frightening themselves with thoughts of drugs, murders, and kidnapping. The U.S. Department of State (**www.travel.state.gov**) maintains a list of travel warnings about foreign countries, and the one about Colombia, posted as of September 2005, would scare anyone.

> *The Department of State warns U.S. citizens of the dangers of travel to Colombia. Violence by narcoterrorist groups and other criminal elements continues to affect all parts of the country, urban and rural, and border areas. Citizens of the United States and other countries continue to be the victims of threats, kidnappings, and other violence...*

And that was just for starters.

I had a nice chat with the guy, but I did not hear back from him. As 2005 wore on, however, I became aware that regardless of what the Department of State said, or what the average American thinks, lots of people go to Colombia from the United States for medical care and plastic surgery without worrying much or at all about crime. Mostly they are Colombian-Americans, true. But Colombia is also in a position to court medical tourists, and is doing so successfully. Yes, Colombia has a big image problem to overcome in the United States, and I can not quite bring myself to suggest to anyone that Colombia would be near the top of my list of recommended destinations for medical tourists. But, still, people go. Everyday life in Colombia is not what we might imagine it to be, based on news reports and official warnings.

I say this as an example and stark reminder to inexperienced international travelers that much of the world is not what we read about in headlines. There are no stern warnings from the Department of State about most countries to rival that of the one about Colombia, but there are cautions about crime, sickness, political upheaval, and possible natural disasters for just about every country on the planet. Take them into account, certainly, but remember that millions of "average Americans" do travel internationally every year without incident. For contrast, I'll close with what the Australian government tells its citizens who are thinking of visiting the United States:

> The United States is subject to a wide range of natural hazards including tsunamis, volcanoes, and earthquake activity around the Pacific Basin; hurricanes along the Atlantic and Gulf of Mexico coasts; tornadoes in the midwest and southeast; mud slides in California; forest fires in the west; and flooding. In the event of a natural disaster, local authorities will provide advice.

I chuckled, when I first read that. Looking back at it, after Hurricane Katrina decimated New Orleans and the Gulf coast, I wondered about relative levels of safety around the world for travelers. I do know that I have a sense of my own strangeness when visiting a foreign country for the first time; but I have yet to feel any less safe than I ever have in any U.S. city.

CHAPTER 7

Brazil: State of the Art in Aesthetic Makeovers

No country has given more to the development of medical tourism and to cosmetic surgery, or has received less in return financially, than Brazil. The balance, however, is being redressed. Cosmetic surgery may not have been invented in Brazil, but thanks to Ivo Pitanguy, M.D., it may as well have been. He has flamboyantly led the way for mass acceptance of surgery for beauty purposes, while training and sending back to the rest of the world some of its most respected and creative surgeons—more than 500 of them, at last count.

"It's almost like he's a brand," Christi de Moraes told me, sitting outside an Orlando hotel late on a Sunday morning in May 2005. Sitting next to her, Fabio Zamprogno, M.D., a plastic surgeon from Vitória, Brazil, nodded. We had talked about Dr. Pitanguy's status as a Brazilian national icon. "He is just Pitanguy to us," he said. "Everyone in Brazil knows who he is."

The two, along with a coterie of volunteers, were in Orlando for the second annual convention of MedNetBrazil (www.mednetbrazil.com), the company de Moraes had started 2 years earlier. MedNetBrazil has its roots in her own experience. She wanted to help other people safely and affordably do what she had done herself—have weight-loss surgery (WLS), leave obesity behind, and, later, undergo a full-body makeover. She was among the first of Dr. Zamprogno's "FrankenBarbies," a term laughingly coined by another of his patients, Linda Giangreco of California, who was also in Orlando helping.

"FRANKENBARBIES"—THE ULTIMATE

Christi and Linda are both beautiful and petite now, and it is hard to imagine either of them at more than 300 pounds, which they both were a few years back before having weight-loss surgery. But they weren't FrankenBarbies until after Dr. Zamprogno had finished with them. This is no slur on his skills—rather the opposite. Christi and Linda, after losing more than 180 pounds each, both still had the legacy, the reminder of their old selves, in the form of hanging rolls and folds of skin that had encased their former bulk. It was Dr. Zamprogno—Dr. Fabio as his patients usually call him—who excised the skin, shaped their new legs, stomachs, butts, torsos, necks, even faces, leaving as little scarring as he could manage.

They are his FrankenBarbies, as close as he could make them to what they had always physically wanted to be. A full-body makeover on a post-WLS patient is about as extreme as an aesthetic makeover can get. In the first 2 years that Dr. Fabio has been doing the surgeries, he has sculpted more than a hundred FrankenBarbies from the United States, and several FrankenKens as well.

"It's not just a humorous throw-away line," Linda said to me later, when I asked her if she minded if I credited her with coining the word FrankenBarbies. "It's an important reference to the amazing transformation that takes place immediately after reconstructive surgery."

In fact, what occurs is quite the opposite from a Frankenstein-like outcome. "It's exactly like waking up and finding that Dr. Fabio has turned you from an unsightly mess, with body parts in disarray, sagging and bagging, into a princess with all the right parts in all the right places," she says. "The immediacy of the results is apparent even through the swelling, bruising, stitches, and bandages. It takes a bit of time, 5 minutes at least, for you to wrap your mind around a change that you previously thought impossible."

> It's exactly like waking up and finding that Dr. Fabio has turned you from an unsightly mess, with body parts in disarray, sagging and bagging, into a princess with all the right parts in all the right places.

The MedNetBrazil convention brought more than 40 past and future FrankenBarbies and FrankenKens to Orlando. It was a frantic, 3-day love fest. The patients adore their surgeons and Christi for making their transformations possible, and they return the feeling. There was a bit of a Carnaval feeling in the air; one could not help but think Ivo Pitanguy would have enjoyed the weekend.

THE NAME IS PITANGUY

The Pitanguy brand in plastic surgery is unassailable, and that is the number-one advantage Christi, Dr. Fabio, and all of Brazil have as they compete for medical-tourism patients and their dollars. Even plastic surgeons in the United States who are ferociously

> If you want to go to Dr. Pitanguy, or someone trained by Dr. Pitanguy, no one will argue. Rumor has it that Dr. Pitanguy did Sophia Loren's work.

dead set against the idea of patients traveling abroad for procedures pull up short when Dr. Pitanguy is mentioned. The implication is that, well—he's different. If you want to go to Dr. Pitanguy, or someone trained by Dr. Pitanguy, no one will argue. The rumor for years has been that Dr. Pitanguy did Sophia Loren's work. Who is going to argue?

Ironically, however, the very success of Dr. Pitanguy in popularizing cosmetic surgery in Brazil and in training surgeons from around the world has, in some ways, kept Brazilian surgeons from taking a lead in the medical-tourism marketplace. Though some American jet-setters came to Dr. Pitanguy, there was no need to make a point of going after the U.S. market, as surgeons have done in other countries. Why bother, when there are 180 million Brazilians, and they all seem to want plastic surgery?

I joked with Dr. Fabio that Brazilian doctors must have finally run out of Brazilians to operate on—hasn't everyone there already had plastic surgery? He grinned, "It is not quite like that." But perhaps it is getting that way, a little. There are 4,400 plastic surgeons in Brazil, and they have been very busy for years. In Brazil, aesthetic surgeons have succeeded, among other things, in making surgery both accessible and affordable for the general population, more so than anywhere else in the world.

"Cheap surgery," viewed with such suspicion in the United States, is commonplace. Top international surgeons command as much for procedures as any of the top surgeons in the United States, but the prices of many Brazilian surgeons are within the reach of the working poor. There are even free clinics for the poor.

AN ABUNDANCE OF TALENT

I asked Christi and Dr. Fabio whether there was a quality problem in Brazil with cut-rate surgeons, perhaps ones who are not board-certified. Dr. Fabio seemed genuinely puzzled by the question. A bemused Christi explained to him: "In other countries, even in the United States, doctors who are not board-certified in plastic surgery often do cosmetic procedures."

His face cleared: "In Vitória [a city of about 300,000], there are 104 plastic surgeons," he said. "There are so many board-certified plastic surgeons, there is no place for someone who does not have the medical background. If there is someone who did not do his resident training in plastic surgery, there are no patients for him. There is no market in Brazil for a doctor who is not qualified."

> "There is no market in Brazil for a doctor who is not qualified."

But few Brazilian surgeons have aggressively gone after the international market. In particular, they have not pursued the vastly expanded market for plastic surgery that has developed in the United States in the past 10 to 15 years.

It's not that surgeons are not interested in foreign business; it is that Brazil does not have the infrastructure to receive patients, says Dr. Fabio. "The patients come from Italy, from Switzerland, from France, from England ... and some come from the United States. But usually, they have some family in Brazil who will house them."

In Vitória, at least, MedNetBrazil's medical-tourism clients—many of them Dr. Fabio's patients—have the option of staying at a luxurious spa instead of a hotel. The company is working on agreements with other doctors and other facilities in other Brazilian cities that will give medical tourists a full range of choices in surgeons, locations, and accommodations.

Her company is certainly not the only one to offer such medical "concierge" services to foreigners, but Christi was among the first to recognize that many more people from the United States would come to Brazil for medical care and plastic surgery if they knew about it and if it was easier to do. MedNetBrazil has accomplished that, using the Internet for marketing and for hand-holding patients throughout the process.

Competitors in Brazil are popping up left and right now, and nascent U.S.-based medical-tourism companies are entering the fray. But Christi de Moraes is in the right place at the right time—with a head start. If you could create the perfect person to start up a successful medical-tourism business in Brazil, she would be it. She was born in the United States where she started in the hospitality industry. She married a Brazilian, and she speaks fluent Portuguese. She's also been through the medical system in both the United States and Brazil as a patient and has emerged a FrankenBarbie with a passion for what she does.

"Everything in my life has led me to this," she says. "There is no doubt in my mind that I am doing what my destiny called me to do."

FOR MEDICAL TOURISM, A WORLD OF POTENTIAL

One would think that Brazil, by reason of its outstanding reputation for aesthetic surgery, would be similarly poised to cash in on medical tourism. Many surgeons want the business from the United States and other countries, but only a few have gone after it.

Many are just now figuring out how to market their services internationally. More and more Brazilian surgeons are following Dr. Pitanguy's lead. Surgeons are putting up Web sites in English, affiliating themselves with businesses that can send patients from outside the country, and reaching out through the Internet by setting up online forums and even doing online video consultations.

In-country cosmetic surgery has long been affordable for any Brazilian, and it has long been sought after by the wealthy elites of the West, but increasingly, it is a viable option to consider for the average North American or European who wants quality work at a substantially lower price than available at home. Brazilian dentists, ophthalmologists, and gastrointestinal surgeons are also competing, or are poised to compete, for patients from abroad.

THE BRAZIL OPTION

You can look farther south to Argentina, or you can look to Venezuela. You can look to Chile, to Peru, even to Colombia and the smaller countries of South America and find outstanding plastic surgeons with modest prices, but it is Brazil that has the most potential as a medical-tourism destination.

There are very good reasons why—despite the reputation of its surgeons—Brazil is currently better known for exporting cosmetic techniques, training aesthetic surgeons from abroad, and for the physical beauty of its own citizens, rather than as a destination for North Americans of average means looking for an alternative to high surgery prices.

The Language Barrier

The official language of Brazil is **Portuguese**, and it is the language that Brazilians proudly use. Certainly many educated Brazilians speak English, Spanish, or other languages. But outside of the top international surgeons in the hub cities of Rio de Janeiro and São Paulo, there are as yet few surgeons who are accustomed to having English-speaking patients and marketing to the English-speaking world. According to Dr. Fabio, since they don't have the language capability, Brazilian plastic surgeons would rather turn patients away than have them come and not experience great care.

> Doctors would rather turn patients away than have them come and not experience great care.

Geography

São Paulo is an **8-hour flight from Miami**. While the trip to Brazil is certainly less daunting for most prospective medical tourists from the United States than traveling to Thailand, Malaysia, or India would be, it's still more of a challenge than going to Mexico, Costa Rica, or Santo Domingo—where, ironically, you can find Pitanguy-trained surgeons who look to the United States for patients.

Infrastructure

With notable exceptions, Brazilian surgeons are only just starting to do what they must do to cater to a broader international market for cosmetic surgery. Plastic-surgery patients are not typical tourists; they are patients, first and foremost, and want to be cared for as such.

Marketing

Aside from Dr. Pitanguy and a few other surgeons who have cultivated international reputations and clienteles, Brazilian surgeons have started attracting patients through Internet marketing, personal trips to the United States to meet prospective patients, and affiliating themselves with medical tourism companies, travel firms, and concierge services. It is not unfair to say that the marketing of Brazil as a destination for prospective plastic-surgery patients, until perhaps 2003, relied almost totally on the reputation of its surgeons, the renown of the **Pitanguy Institute**, occasional stories in the mass media, and, always, word-of-mouth.

MedNetBrazil, as a business, and Dr. Fabio, as a surgeon, have been pioneers in marketing directly to the broader North American market. I have chosen them carefully as examples, though they are not the only resources available and more are coming online all the time.

HOW TO FIND A SURGEON

You could simply show up in **São Paulo**, **Rio de Janeiro**, **Vitória**, **Curitiba**, or any major coastal city in Brazil, unannounced, check into an upscale hotel that caters to tourists, and ask at the front desk if there are any good, inexpensive plastic surgeons nearby who speak English and take walk-ins. I have heard of people who, more or less, have done just that—gone to Brazil on vacation and come back with a face-lift.

It may sound reckless and cavalier, but people do such things, and there are reputable plastic surgeons who are willing to accommodate them. Just because I wouldn't do it, or just because some doctors and surgeons would be deeply disturbed at the suggestion that someone

> It may sound reckless and cavalier, but people are known to show up for plastic surgery as walk-in patients.

might have plastic surgery on a "whim," doesn't mean it's wrong for everyone.

Nevertheless, in so doing, you should exercise every reasonable precaution about choosing a qualified surgeon in a compressed time frame. You also should consider the possibility that you will have to extend your stay in Brazil to allow for the possibility of slow healing or complications.

On the upside, by just showing up, you may have access to more prospective surgeons than you would if you were trying to find a surgeon via the Internet or even by phone. Plus, you would get to talk to them face-to-face.

On the downside, you might not find a suitable surgeon at all, or you might not be able to get your procedure scheduled to suit your time frame. "Just go and figure it out" is an option, and not as ridiculous as it might sound. This presumes that you are planning to go to Brazil anyway, and that you're willing to go home without having surgery if you are not fortunate enough to find a qualified surgeon who can do what you want in a time frame acceptable to you. There are very few other places in the world where this might be a reasonable plan, even for the small number of people who are willing to give it a try.

Limited but Growing Resources Online

The second way to find a suitable plastic surgeon in Brazil is to research your choice from afar, via the Internet, e-mail, and telephone, as described in chapter 5. There are still relatively few resources available in English, and the search for Brazilian surgeons has been complicated by the fact that www.sbcp.org, a site supposedly sponsored by the Brazilian Society of Plastic Surgeons is, in fact, not owned or maintained by the society! The valid site for the society is **www.cirurgiaplastica.org.br.**

The site is fully functional with the Microsoft Internet Explorer Web browser. Though it is in Portuguese, you can probably maneuver enough to check things like whether a surgeon is a member. There is a scarcity of truly useable English sites for Brazil, so the following might help get you started in your search.

- The best Brazilian Web site with an English-language version is, perhaps unsurprisingly, that of the **Pitanguy Institute (www.pitanguy.com)**. The Pitanguy Clinic, however, is not a low-budget option for foreigners. Prices are comparable to those in the United States, presumably due to the institute's reputation.
- **The International Society of Aesthetic Plastic Surgery (ISAPS)** at **www.isaps.org** offers contact information on more than 150 Brazilian aesthetic surgeons who are members of this society and presumably among the country's elite. Some list Web sites as well as e-mail addresses and phone numbers. Some of the Web sites are in English.
- There are several excellent Yahoo groups that are run for patients and prospective patients by concierge services and/or Brazilian doctors, both for plastic surgery and for bariatric (weight-loss) surgery. See **www.groups.yahoo.com** and search for plastic surgery. Specific group addresses for pages of interest include:

  - **www.health.groups.yahoo.com/group/mednet_brazil**
  - **www.health.groups.yahoo.com/group/drfabiozamprogno plasticsurgeryinBrazil**
  - **www.groups.yahoo.com/group/DrCavalcanti**

- If you do not have the inclination to research exhaustively, but you've decided that Brazil is where you want to go for surgery, take a close look at **concierge services and medical-tourism companies**, as referenced in chapter 5. **MedNetBrazil** is one such company, and most services are relatively new. The merits of using their services are discussed extensively in the Yahoo groups, and in the various support forums on the Web.
- Another firm that made it onto my radar enough to warrant a look is

Cosmetic Vacations (www.cosmeticvacations.com). The company has affiliated itself with several well-known surgeons and facilities in Rio de Janeiro. Two ex-investment bankers started Cosmetic Vacations in early 2004.

"Brazil was always our number-one pick as a country for cosmetic surgery," co-founder Peter Ryan says. "The quality of the surgery and the after-care facilities were known to be of a very high standard. While absolute costs in some other lesser-developed countries were lower than those generated by our pricing model, we felt the quality/price ratio favored Brazil.

> Brazil has every level and type of beauty-related service one can imagine.

"As far as consumer choice is concerned, we believe Brazil offers the most comprehensive array of cosmetic-enhancement services. This is largely a function of local demand—Brazil has every level and type of beauty-related services one can imagine," he adds.

THE COUNTRY

Brazil is the **largest of the Latin American countries**, covering nearly half of the continent of South America. It is the **fifth largest country in the world** after the Russian Federation, Canada, China, and the United States. The Equator passes through the north of the country near Macapá; the Tropic of Capricorn passes through the south near São Paulo. It was claimed by Portugal in the late 1400s, and the first permanent European settlements were founded in the 1530s. Brazil proclaimed independence from Portugal and declared itself under the rule of an emperor in 1822. It became a republic after the abolition of slavery in 1888. More recently, Brazil was under military rule from 1964 until 1985, after which democracy was restored.

Rio de Janeiro and São Paulo are two of the world's great metropolises. They and nine other cities have more than a million inhabitants each. **Brazilians are one of the most ethnically diverse people in the world:** In the extreme south, German and Italian immigration has left distinctive European features. São Paulo has the world's largest Japanese community outside Japan. There's a large black population concentrated in Rio and Salvador.

Rapid industrialization since World War II made Brazil one of the world's ten largest economies, but the distribution of wealth is profoundly uneven. Brazil has grinding poverty amidst its wealth. The cities are dotted with shantytowns.

TOURIST INFORMATION

There are many English-language Web sites devoted to general tourism in Brazil. **Carnaval is one of the biggest international celebrations in the world, the beaches are as renowned as the plastic surgeons, and the culture is rich and varied.** Among the best sites:

- **www.gringoes.com**
- **www.braziltourism.org**
- **www.ipanema.com**
- **www.braziltour.com**

CHAPTER 8

Costa Rica: The Beverly Hills of Central America?

Costa Rica was discovered by Christopher Columbus himself, on his fourth and last trip to the New World in 1502. There were already people living there, of course, but they were especially vulnerable to smallpox, which the Spaniards inadvertently introduced to the region. So most of the natives died or fled. In June of 2005, Costa Ricans who depend on medical tourism for their livelihood were awaiting a different sort of discovery—they were going to be on U.S. network television. And while they didn't expect to be wiped out by the exposure, they were more than a little worried.

A reporter from ABC's *20/20*, Deborah Roberts, and a camera crew had been there the previous fall, 9 long months before. They had followed three American women through their experiences of going to Costa Rica for cosmetic surgery, dogged their every step, actually, in the way that good and thorough TV journalists do, to the point where you wonder— *Would this happen the same way if they weren't there?* What TV does is not passive observation. Whatever happens is, in some sense…produced.

Everyone I know at all well in Costa Rica remembers something about what went on when *20/20* came to town. They remembered Tammy from Georgia and the sisters from Tennessee, Linda and Lori. The three women discovered Costa Rica and its lower-priced plastic surgeons on the Internet, checked their surgeon's credentials online, and participated in online forums. Tammy had a tummy tuck, liposuction, a breast lift and augmentation, and eyelid surgery with Federico Macaya, M.D. Lori, who had previously lost 119 pounds after gastric bypass surgery, had a thigh lift, a tummy tuck, an arm lift, and a breast lift with implants. Her sister Linda had a tummy tuck, liposuction, and breast augmentation. The sisters went to Luis Da Cruz, M.D. All three stayed at Las Cumbres Inn Surgical Retreat, which is also where I spent my first three nights in Costa Rica.

The women had their surgeries and went home. The *20/20* crew got its story—whatever it was—and they went home, too. In Costa Rica, the surgeons, doctors, owners of recovery retreats for patients, hospital staffers, and tourism officials…well, they went on with what they were doing, unobserved, and settled down to wait, wondering what they had gotten themselves into.

By spring, stories were starting to spread. Tammy had complications. There were comments and rumors posted on Internet forums and in e-mails that, in effect, the women were not happy with their cosmetic results, and that it was in part their own faults. They had not followed their recovery plans and had tried to do too much, too soon after surgery. They were smokers and didn't tell their surgeons. Smoking is a taboo for cosmetic surgery patients and is associated with poor healing. The *20/20* segment on Costa Rica was supposed to air in April but was postponed. People in the United States who were curious about what the show would be like—such as other patients and medical tourism business opera-tors—began to wonder in Internet forums if the show would be a "hatchet job," one that might injure the reputation Costa Rican surgeons had worked for decades to build.

April came and went, as did May. I was in Costa Rica in June when *20/20* finally announced that the segment was going to air. "They seemed very nice when they were here," Elke Arends, the proprietress of Las Cumbres, said to me as we sat in the large common room of her inn. "They asked good questions. But you don't know how they are going to show it." She asked me what I thought would happen. I murmured some hopeful things about *20/20*'s reputation; I mean, Barbara Walters and all. Maybe it wouldn't be too bad, I said.

Everyone wanted to know, and most wouldn't be able to watch. ABC wasn't part of the basic cable package in San José. I promised I'd tape it on June 24 back in Connecticut and let them know what I thought.

And back home, it really didn't look good to me, especially from the promotional lead up to the segment. This wasn't about medical tourism at all; it was the "first of seven hours on the 'Seven Deadly Sins,'" ABC's John Stoessel intoned. "And we are starting with pride," and its "extreme example, vanity"…and a woman "so desperate to get her pre-baby body back that she's willing to risk cosmetic surgery at bargain-basement prices." I said some very bad words and prepared for a long hour. What was I going to tell Elke and my dentists, Telma and Josef?

The segment itself was not nearly as negative as the promo had hinted, or as anyone had feared. Tammy did have significant post-surgery complications, but *20/20* noted that she had a history of them. A New York City surgeon was consulted who was openly critical of Dr. Macaya's work, but Macaya was given the opportunity to defend himself. In the end, Tammy told an incredulous Deborah Roberts that she might well return to Costa Rica for follow-up surgery, a revision, if necessary, rather than go to a surgeon in the United States. "I can't financially," she said, when asked straight-out as to why she wouldn't go to a U.S. surgeon. "I have no guarantee that if I spent $25,000 in the United States to do it, it wouldn't have gone wrong as well." She was pleased, in particular, with the eye work Dr. Macaya had done. Lori and Linda were mostly happy with their results at the hands of Dr. Da Cruz.

I wrote Elke that the show had been presented skeptically, as opposed to negatively. I did not think it would do any harm.

My phone rang the next evening. It was Elke from Costa Rica. She had listened to the show, patched in over a telephone line from the United States. In the 24 hours since the *20/20* segment had aired, more than a thousand people had written to her requesting

> In the 24 hours after the *20/20* segment aired, more than 1,000 people wrote to the Inn seeking information about getting plastic surgery in Costa Rica.

information about going to Costa Rica for surgery. "Jeff, what are we going to do with them all?" she asked. Las Cumbres can handle perhaps 20, at any given time. But Elke was pretty happy. Some weeks after, I started seeing some grumbling online about how Dr. Da Cruz was not responding to e-mails as promptly as he once had. The speculation was that he had gotten very busy, indeed.

The *20/20* segment was presented online under the headline: "Is It Wise to Hunt for Cut-Rate Plastic Surgery?" The answer from the patients could be summed up as, "Worked for me!"

IT WORKED FOR ME!

Costa Rica is where I went for my own dental work, of course, and I can therefore recommend it based on my own experience. I could make this chapter a sort of love letter to my excellent dentists, to the surgeons I've met, and to all the people who treated me so kindly. But I'm just one guy and again, I will tell you that my word alone is insufficient. I can tell you what I know, what I saw, and what I heard.

I can also tell you that Costa Rica is not for everyone any more than is any other country. Even now, when people write and ask me about my own dental work (*Are you still happy with your choice? Would you do it again?*), I respond that, yes, I'm thrilled, and I would do it again. But there are other dentists in Costa Rica, other dentists in other countries. Shop around. Do your own homework. I am quite sure that my dentists have glowing references from patients who advise anyone and everyone that Prisma Dental is the best and only place to go.

> The Costa Rican medical community has been in the medical tourism business since the late 1970s.

The Costa Rican medical community has been in the medical tourism business a long time, since the late 1970s or early 1980s, at least. Experience helps.

In Costa Rica, there is such a thing as a "typical" medical tourism experience. "Nice trip, pretty uneventful. I'm still healing but I've come a long way in a short amount of time," is how Lori Smith of Florida described her trip in September 2005. She went with her husband and they stayed at the Martino Resort & Spa, in Alajuela, near both the airport and San José. Lori had her upper and lower eyes done, and some work on her nose. The surgery and hospital fees were $2,100, and she estimated that she and her husband spent about $1,400 on the accommodations, meals, and incidental expenses. The Martino Resort & Spa is a small, five-star hotel, pricier than most of the other recovery retreats around San José. Add airfare, and Lori's cost for the facial cosmetic surgery and a week at a resort with her husband cost in the neighborhood of $4,000. She says she was quoted $5,000 for the surgery alone in Florida. Many people who go abroad for surgery have more expensive procedures, stay at less expensive places, and count much higher savings. The more publicized cases of extreme makeovers in faraway lands for tens of thousands of dollars less than U.S. prices are by no means the rule. Even for relatively minor procedures and comparatively small savings, people like the Smiths are going to Costa Rica because of the reputation of the island's surgeons, doctors, dentists, recovery retreats, resorts, and spas.

Costa Rica is really on its second generation of cosmetic surgeons that has built practices by looking to North America for patients. Arnoldo Fournier, M.D., who was Lori Smith's surgeon, and Dr. Macaya, on the hot seat with *20/20* in 2005, were among the first to recognize and capitalize on the possibilities of medical tourism in the 1970s and 1980s. The Rosenstock-Lieberman Center for Cosmetic Plastic Surgery has been in business 25 years. In fact, Costa Rica earned its nickname in the world of cosmetic surgery as the "Beverly Hills of Central America" because its medical community is well established as are its facilities.

Costa Rican medical tourism did not grow up around a central medical facility, and was not guided or funded by any prescient business entity or government agency. Even after a decade of spectacular growth, medical tourism in Costa Rica still has the feel of a cottage industry grown to a town where everyone knows everyone else, or are even related by blood or marriage. Newcomer physicians are scrutinized and are either welcomed or found wanting by informal peer review and consensus, which is part of why the general quality of the patient experience has been maintained. Ruben Martin, who, with his wife, Lorena, runs the CheTica Ranch Medical Recovery Center in the hills above San José, told me of a surgeon who had disappointed a few patients. Nothing life-threatening was involved, but there had been disappointments."If people asked, we could not recommend him," Ruben said. "How could we when there are others who are so good?"

RECOVERY RETREATS

Recovery retreats such as CheTica and Las Cumbres Inn have functioned for years as gateways for medical tourism in Costa Rica. They try to avoid recommending specific surgeons or doctors to prospective patients—*it's the patient's responsibility to choose* is the view they try to take—but most are affiliated at least unofficially with some favorites. The medical community serves as one safeguard against surgical incompetence, as it does in the United States and elsewhere. People should verify the credentials and board certification of their doctors. The online patient community, where experiences both good and bad are shared, serves as another check. If a prospective patient sticks with a short list of those surgeons, doctors, and dentists who have at least the unofficial seal of approval from a recovery retreat of longstanding reputation, he or she is likely to have an "uneventful" medical tourism experience.

On my first trip to Costa Rica, I observed that patients who wanted to be insulated from just about anything that would smack of culture shock could do so by sticking with the established recovery retreat routine. If you can manage to coordinate booking dates with a surgeon, a recovery retreat, and an airline, you can concentrate pretty much on your surgery and recovery. You'll be met at the airport by someone who speaks English. You'll be shuttled to and from your medical appointments. You'll have choices in accommodations and amenities, minor decisions to make about meals, but you'll be looked after, cared for, and worried about—sheltered and coddled—from the time you arrive until the time you go home. This sums up the "typical" experience of medical tourism, Costa Rica style.

> You'll be shuttled around by someone who speaks English. You'll be sheltered and cared for from the time you arrive until the time you go home.

Of course, this is also a generalization. Everyone is different, and I will fall back again on "do your homework" in researching surgeons and accommodations. Be cautious about accepting a single, glowing recommendation from me or anyone else. I make the broad statements about the Costa Rican experience by good and independently verifiable reason, however. Setting aside my own anecdotal experiences, anyone can go online and find so many first-person accounts of trips to Costa Rica for cosmetic surgery that they would have to come to the same general conclusions that I did. If you spend the time, you will also discern the variety of good individual experiences, and you'll find the bad personal experiences as well. You will find people who disliked where they stayed, hated the food and felt they were treated shabbily or even cheated. You'll find people who were bored, lonely, and/or scared during their stay, who thought every moment of their journey felt alien. You'll find people who were dissatisfied with their surgery results. You'll find angry people who wish they had never heard of Costa Rica—but not many.

And some things simply can't be anticipated. Anyone who expected an entirely unremarkable stay at Las Cumbres Inn on the same week that four New York City exotic dancers were in town for breast augmentation surgery was at least somewhat mistaken. Elke Arends, the owner of Las Cumbres, hesitated a moment and smiled before describing the week as unusually high-spirited. The women chafed a bit at the enforced peace and quiet, and by all accounts were enormously entertaining, though certainly not in the same way that they would have been on the job back in the United States. "They were good girls," Elke finally said, diplomatically, a little surprised that someone in the United States would have heard about a small amount of commotion at her place.

You'll want to consider everything you read, and weigh it all. But even if you decide against going to Costa Rica for cosmetic surgery or other medical treatment, you will have also discovered that of the people who decided to go, a large number, certainly the vast majority, had broadly similar and satisfying trips.

WORD OF MOUTH
In the United States, former patients and, more recently, medical tourism businesses, help keep the customers coming, or even escort them in.

Didi Carr Reuben, of Pacific Palisades, California, went to Costa Rica for
a face-lift in 1997 after hearing about it from a teller in her bank. She had
been working on saving $20,000 for her surgery with a "hotsy totsy Beverly
Hills plastic surgeon," as she puts it on her Web site. Instead, she ended
up in the hands of Alejandro Lev, M.D. The far more inexpensive face-lift
was a success. Someone who disapproves of cosmetic surgery, which I
don't, would say Didi looks almost indecently like her daughter, Gable.
She also had a colonoscopy in Costa Rica in 2002. It cost $400, including
the hospital stay and anesthesiologist—less, she says, than the procedure
would have cost her in the United States even with insurance.

Today, she runs **Didi's Sleepaway Camp For the Terminally Vain
(www.terminallyvain.com)** and Costa Rica is her home away from
home. Didi's puckishly named "camp" runs on an irregular schedule
year-round. A two-week "sleepaway" in Costa Rica, including everything
(air fare from California, recovery retreat accommodations, meals,
face and brow lift package, including hospital fees) cost about $7,300
in 2005. She shepherds patients to San José primarily for Dr. Lev but
also recommends the same dentists who did my teeth, as well as her
own gastroenterologist and a specialist in weight-loss surgery. Her
own expenses are covered by Dr. Lev, but she doesn't run the camp as
a business, preferring that patients make donations to their favorite
charities if they wish. Lev, of course, is the medical professional;
Didi is a fan.

Though Didi is an unabashed booster for Costa Rican medical tourism,
she recognizes that it's not for everyone; her Web site acknowledges
naysayers and she does not take plastic surgery lightly, either. But she
doesn't shy away from comparing the work done by her own surgeon
with what she sees on the faces of women who have had their lifts done
in nearby Beverly Hills, at three or four times the total expense. I asked
her for a West Coast perspective.

"Yes, there's no question about the fact that people see Beverly Hills
as the place to have plastic surgery (if money is not an object, of course),
she responded in an e-mail. "It's funny, but when I go to restaurants in
Beverly Hills I see many women who have had a face-lift and they all

seem to look alike. I don't know why that is, it just is…an observation. The women I see in Beverly Hills seem to be more pulled and tight looking. One woman from Beverly Hills came to me and then to Dr. Lev asking for the pulled and tight Beverly Hills look. Dr. Lev wouldn't do it; he said it distorts the mouth."

Many individual surgeons in Costa Rica have former patients from the United States engaged in bringing in new business; Didi is simply among the more prolific and visible. Others have found, over time, that the growth in medical tourism in Costa Rica has created a substantial business opportunity.

On the other coast, in Garrison, New York, Stephanie Sulger went to Costa Rica for a face-lift in 2002 and started **Medical Tours International (plasticsurgerytravel.com)** soon thereafter, handling referrals and patient services for a number of Costa Rican surgeons and dentists. Sulger, a registered nurse, ironically was still working part-time in operating rooms for U.S. plastic surgeons in 2005.

"It all started after my own face-lift. The referral thing was just a whim," she says, but the business has expanded beyond Costa Rica and beyond cosmetic surgery and dentistry. She is now looking at opportunities in South America and the Far East, and has changed the name of the company to **World Wide Medical Tourism (worldwidemedicaltourism.com)** though she continues with plasticsurgerytravel.com specifically for Costa Rica, where she started.

"One of the really great things about this business is the gratitude I receive from clients," Sulger says, echoing something I have heard over and over again from both overseas surgeons and business people involved in setting up medical tourism trips. "I remember how I felt when I found out about Costa Rica and realized I didn't have to succumb to U.S. surgical costs.

"Since then I have focused on the safety issues involved in going to a foreign country for surgery. I have found their surgical standards of care to be at least as good as here in the states. They use quality control procedures comparable to our JCAHO standards. The hospital nurses almost always have advanced degrees in nursing and are bilingual. The surgeons are all board certified and much more accessible and approachable than many U.S. doctors."

JCAHO is the U.S.-based Joint Commission on Accreditation of Healthcare Organizations, a not-for-profit organization that sets health-care quality standards, primarily in the United States. Overseas hospitals are moving to comply with JCAHO standards in part to reassure patients from the United States that care will be at the level they expect. Most countries with modern health-care facilities already have their own accreditation standards and enforcement, however, and Costa Rica is no exception. When I spoke in June 2005 with Francisco Gólcher, M.D., of the Costa Rican Ministry of Health, he gestured at reams of computer printouts when I asked about accreditation, and we thumbed through them together. "We have extensive standards, comparable to those anywhere. We do the inspections and we do the licensing," he said. "Especially in the last ten years, with the opening of more new hospitals, the quality keeps getting better." In a lengthy interview, Dr. Gólcher spoke proudly of the quality of both the public and private health-care systems in Costa Rica. His department has 81 offices in the country. "We have the people to do the job," he said.

> Overseas hospitals are moving to comply with JCAHO standards in part to reassure patients coming from the United States.

I had reason to write to him again just a month later, when tragedy struck the Costa Rican health-care system. A fire swept through Calderon Guardia Hospital in San José, killing 18. The 62-year-old public hospital had lacked safety measures required under recently implemented national fire regulations—including fire hoses, emergency lighting, and a fire escape. An Associated Press story said the fire raised questions about safety precautions in other medical facilities throughout the Central American country—which was unfair, as it turned out.

"I understand that the media sometimes can assume that when something like this happens, the same situation exists with the rest of our medical facilities," Dr. Gólcher responded. "That was a public hospital and it was old. The private hospitals all have their licenses issued by my office and they are all okay with security and safety issues. The problems are in our oldest public hospital. As you know, we have new public and private hospitals that are well done, very modern."

CIMA HOSPITAL: STATE OF THE ART

CIMA Hospital in the San José suburb of Escazú is the jewel of private health care in Costa Rica. Just five years old, CIMA (Center for International Medicine, though the acronym is from the Spanish name) is run by the International Hospital Corp. (IHC) in Dallas, Texas, which intends to build "the preeminent private health-care system in Latin America, leading the industry in quality, service and profitability." IHC also has CIMA hospitals in Mexico and Brazil. All are **affiliated with Baylor University Medical Center in Texas** under an agreement that permits the CIMA hospitals to send their medical staff and management to participate in Baylor's advanced medical and professional education programs. Baylor also provides consulting support to the CIMA hospitals and their medical staff. All front-line staffers are required to become proficient in English.

"It gives us a certain credibility," Dr. Gólcher observed, and he is right.

CIMA boasts Costa Rica's only licensed helipad, which receives 8-9 landings per year, a medical office building with 99 suites and 180 physicians representing 40 different specialties, and 54 in-patient beds. A second office building is planned, as is an advanced cancer-treatment center. In 2005, CIMA opened the first private psychiatric treatment facility in Central America. In short, CIMA both appears to be and is exactly what anyone in the United States thinks of when they think of a good hospital. Its patients are Costa Ricans who prefer and can afford private health care; the growing number of U.S. citizens who make their homes in Costa Rica; and medical tourists from throughout Central America and the Caribbean and, in small but increasing numbers, from the United States.

CIMA Hospital Services

CIMA offers comprehensive, modern health care and makes a point of making its services known to tourists. It advertises these services:

- 24-hour emergency facilities staffed with both adult and pediatric trauma-certified physicians
- Helipad (Air Ambulance Access)
- 6-bed, fully-monitored and staffed Intensive Care Unit
- Special Shock and Trauma Emergency Room
- 180 qualified physicians (on site, English-speaking) representing over 40 clinical specialties
- Complete imaging services, including High-speed Helical CT scan, Open MRI, nuclear medicine, ultrasound, mammogram, bone-density scan, and conventional X-ray
- Clinical and pathology laboratory services, including blood bank
- 54 fully-equipped, private, modern rooms and luxury suites
- 24-hour on-site pharmacy
- Emergency medical support and transport provided by affiliates throughout Costa Rica

CIMA emphasizes inexpensive prices on:

- Cosmetic and reconstructive plastic surgery
- Oral and dental procedures
- Physical rehabilitation services

For those planning to move to Costa Rica, CIMA markets itself as a complete health-care provider offering:

- A full-service, acute-care hospital, including emergency room and intensive care unit
- Medical check-up plans (executive physicals), tailored to age and specific needs
- Special endoscopic department for complete gastric, intestinal, and colon procedures
- Advanced maternity unit, newborn nursery, and neonatal intensive care unit
- Out-patient surgeries and services
- Physical and respiratory therapy services

And, saving the best for last, as far as many people from the United States are concerned: They accept many insurance plans from the United States and European countries.

Oscar Suárez, M.D., is head of the department of plastic and cosmetic surgery at CIMA. When I showed up at his busy office suite for an interview for this book, the receptionist initially assumed I was a prospective patient and was embarrassed when I said I was not. It was easy to let it go with a rueful smile. For feeling one's age, there's nothing quite like spending a lot of time hanging out with cosmetic surgeons. I resisted the temptation to ask Dr. Suárez if he could do something about the bags under my eyes and instead we talked about CIMA and Costa Rica's place in the world of medical tourism. He looks to be in his late 30s. He trained in Costa Rica and in Mexico and has a distinguished resumé. He visits the U.S. regularly. He paid tribute to the surgeons who kick-started medical tourism in Costa Rica decades ago. Modern facilities such as CIMA allow younger surgeons to build upon the legacy of those who came before him, Dr. Suárez said.

"The older generation—and I personally get along with them very well —is a group of surgeons who, due to the fine work they did, also developed a very good thing for the country," he commented. "But CIMA has made a difference. Even though price-wise it is attractive for people to come here, sometimes—and it is only logical—people are very apprehensive to come because they think they're going out to the 'Third World,' you know? But then when they come here they see that we have these facilities. Someone who comes from, say, Ohio or California can relate. They can look at this hospital and see it as something familiar to them."

Dr. Suárez noted the proliferation of outpatient cosmetic surgical facilities and clinics in the United States and says he fells fortunate to be working in a hospital environment. Operating room charges at CIMA are a small fraction of what they can be in the United States, measured in hundreds of dollars rather than thousands.

"My friends in the United States who are directly associated with hospitals and do their surgeries in hospitals feel they have a very hard time being competitive in the market because of the cost of the hospital. It's outrageous, I think, sometimes. It's very difficult to find surgeons who work in the aesthetic part of plastic surgery who work in hospital environments. I was asked several times to associate with clinics. I'd think about it, and then I'd get this empty feeling that I'd be there all alone. If there are any kinds of complications, I would really like to have the support of a hospital behind me."

ROSENSTOCK-LIEBERMAN CENTER

When Dr. Suárez talks about the older generation it is another reminder that the Costa Rican medical community, though growing, remains small enough that it is not much of a stretch to think of it as an extended family. Sometimes, this is literally true. When I mentioned to my dentist, Telma, that I might be a candidate for corrective eye surgery, she was able to recommend her older brother, an ophthalmologist. And at the **Rosenstock-Lieberman Center for Cosmetic Plastic Surgery**, the "next generation" of cosmetic surgeons is a son and a son-in-law of the center's founders, Noe Rosenstock, M.D., and Clara Lieberman, M.D. Joseph Cohen, M.D., married into the family. Otherwise, perhaps, he'd be practicing in the United States, where he attended the University of the Pacific in California as an undergraduate and, later, did his residency in general surgery at Easton Hospital in Pennsylvania. Both he and his brother-in-law, Rashi Rosenstock, M.D., maintain memberships in medical associations in the United States, as do many of the more prominent Costa Rican cosmetic surgeons. Rashi Rosenstock did his residency at the prestigious Pitanguy Institute in Brazil.

Though Dr. Suárez is more comfortable in the environs of a hospital, surgeons who work in their own well-equipped facilities note that there is no data that suggests that there is a difference in safety. The Rosenstock center has two state-of-the-art operating rooms. The décor of the reception area is understated, the art on the walls, tasteful. Dr. Cohen's office, however, reflects more the pace of the busy facility. His work is strewn on his desk around a computer on which he handles most of the center's patient contact via e-mail. The walls are covered with photos of dozens of patients, both pre- and post-operative. He is low-key about discussing the center. Earlier, I had been told by a friend to expect that this would be so—that the Rosenstocks and Liebermans are sensitive to their standing in the larger medical community, a little embarrassed to be singled out by the media on a regular basis. But he talks easily about Costa Rican medical care and plastic surgery.

"They come for the price, of course," Dr. Cohen says of patients from abroad. "But they come back again for the quality. Our costs are much lower than in the States." So, we mostly talked about things I already knew and speculated on how Costa Rica's medical system might handle continued explosive growth in medical tourism. Costa Rica is small. Skilled surgeons do not become so overnight. Growth could be a problem, Dr. Cohen acknowledged. But not yet. Costa Rican universities continue to turn out doctors, nurses, and health professionals. According to Dr.

> "They come for the price, of course, but they come back again for the quality."

Gólcher of the Ministry of Health, the country actually has unemployment in the medical sector, despite growth in the economy. New hospitals and medical facilities are planned. Until relatively recently, it has been a challenge for Costa Rica and other developing countries to hold onto their trained professionals, including in the medical field. With economic growth has come more opportunity locally. There is room for further growth, especially with continued investment from abroad.

INSIDE COSTA RICA
Aside from the quality and availability of medical care, Costa Rica, generally, is unrelentingly hospitable to foreigners. **Tourism is the country's No. 1 industry**, having surpassed agricultural production in the last decade. More than 1.5 million visitors from abroad entered the country in 2005, mostly for beach vacations and adventure or eco-tourism.

The Language Barrier
The national language is **Spanish**. English is spoken widely wherever tourists are found, but don't make the assumption that everyone speaks

English, or that those who do speak or understand it perfectly. Even for those who speak Spanish well or fluently, **the local dialect, Tico**, may provide some challenges.

Certainly, surgeons, doctors, and dentists who market services to patients abroad are **accustomed to doing business in English**, as are front-line staff members of recovery retreats, resorts, and hotels. As with traveling anywhere and dealing with strangers, however, it's advisable to take a little extra care communicating to make sure you understand and are understood, especially in medical or travel matters.

Geography

Costa Rica is a country about the **size of West Virginia**. It is bordered by Panama to the southeast, Nicaragua to the north, the Pacific Ocean to the south and west, and the Caribbean to the east. San José International Airport is about a 2-hour direct flight from Miami, 3 hours from Dallas, 5 from New York, and approximately 7 from Los Angeles. Roughly half of the country's population of about 4 million lives in the elevated **Central Valley** area, where the capital, **San José**, is. Though tropical, the Central Valley is high enough (3,000 feet above sea level) that **temperatures remain in the 70s and 80s (Fahrenheit) most of the time**. The dry season is from December to April.

Infrastructure

As mentioned earlier, Costa Rican surgeons, doctors, and dentists have been in the medical tourism business for a long time. Nervous or inexperienced medical tourists are best off sticking with the recommendations of whichever professional they select, or working with a medical tourism company or directly with a resort or recovery retreat. The best-known recovery retreats all have distinctive characters (and pricing). Looking online, you'll find they all have their adherents. I have stayed at both CheTica Ranch (**www.cheticaranch.com**) and Las Cumbres Inn (**www.lascumbresinn.com**) and enjoyed both enormously. However, there are at least a half-dozen others that are prominent and new ones are opening to meet growing demand.

Marketing

There are a number of large Web sites extolling the virtue of medical and health tourism in Costa Rica, and many surgeons, doctors, and dentists maintain their own sites and advertise online. In my experience, Costa Rica is the easiest country mentioned in this book on which to do research on medical tourism. In fact, it was a contributing factor in my decision to go there. There is a wealth of information online and it was, and is, relatively easy to find. Search for "Costa Rica" and whatever medical specialty in which you're interested. Pay attention to the related ads.

HOW TO FIND A SURGEON

Even though it is easy to find marketing information about Costa Rica and Costa Rican cosmetic surgeons, doctors, and dentists, there is, as of this writing, no comprehensive site for the professional association of plastic and cosmetic surgeons in Costa Rica. Perhaps it is because the organization is small. Yet board-certified surgeons with whom I spoke all voiced varying degrees of concern about less-qualified Costa Rican doctors performing cosmetic procedures. As in other countries, including the United States, any doctor is legally allowed to perform most cosmetic procedures. One would think that the Costa Rican board-certified surgeons would band together at least to the extent of sponsoring an authoritative English-language Web site on which prospective patients could check professional credentials. That may be in the works, I am told.

The best Costa Rican surgeons respect each other, but one gets the impression that they are used to going it mostly alone in business, and used to competing with each other—not together against whole other countries. However, there is a Spanish-language Web site for the **Colegio de Médicos y Cirujanos de Costa Rica (CMC; College of Doctors and Surgeons of Costa Rica) at www.medicos.sa.cr**, where you can check membership.

That said, the top Costa Rican surgeons are easy to find online, either by direct search of the Web as described in Chapter 5, through medical tourism company Web sites, or through recovery retreat sites. It is not ten minutes work to find a half-dozen board-certified surgeons whom a prospective patient can contact.

GETTING AROUND THE COUNTRY

Besides having great weather, San José has a lovely view of **volcanic mountains**, and the city is built close to the ground out of a healthy respect for the region's seismic activity. There are active volcanoes, though they are mostly tourist attractions; none has had a recent eruption of the sort that would alarm anyone. The last major earthquake was in 1991. It primarily affected the eastern part of the country, though there was some damage to buildings and infrastructure in San José.

Besides being a tourist magnet, Costa Rica is **perhaps best known as being the oldest and most stable democracy in Central America, and for having maintained an abiding friendship with the United States** through some fairly tense times in the region.

San José

San José is a big city, with big city amenities and some typical big city problems—crime and traffic being the main ones. Neither should especially concern medical tourists staying at recovery retreats or resorts, all of which are either secure or removed from the city. Unless you go off exploring on your own, all that you'll see of the city will be through the window of a minivan. You'll notice that buildings are gated downtown and windows barred. But if you do get out and about—assuming your medical condition allows it—no extraordinary precautions are required. I enjoyed downtown San José and walked everywhere, though taxi service is reliable and inexpensive.

The city looks prosperous, and has pride and dynamism. There is certainly poverty in Costa Rica, but it is mostly invisible to a tourist in San José. Late one Friday night on my first visit, I was in the back seat of my dentists' SUV, high in the hills overlooking the city lights. Josef was driving, Telma dozing beside him. We had a late dinner but Josef wanted me to see a little more of the country than I had. "We are little," he said, maneuvering down switchbacks and showing me where the local workers of San José live. It was a neighborhood of very small homes—dark, neat, and quiet after 11:00 p.m. "But we have done well. As you can see, our stores, our life is not so different from in the United States. We do not have so much, but Costa Ricans want much the same things as do people in the United States."

Yes, they are little, but how big can they get? How will it change, as this country prospers? I met with officials from the Costa Rican Investment Board (CINDE) the non-profit organization responsible for stimulating direct foreign investment in the country, and asked them. CINDE has primarily been involved in bringing manufacturing companies and jobs to Costa Rica—electronics and medical devices are two notable areas of success.

"What about medical services?" I asked. "What's going on with that?" Heads nodded around the table. It is just beginning, they said.

CHAPTER 9

Mexico: Going South of the Border

Mexico is without doubt the No. 1 destination for thousands of U.S. citizens looking for inexpensive cosmetic surgery, dental care, and alternative health treatments, if for no other reason than proximity. In all, more than 15 million U.S. citizens head south of the border annually, according to the U.S. Department of State.

Yet it doesn't make most short lists of countries that are likely to capitalize on medical tourism, so for months I really didn't know what to say about Mexico in this book. For one thing, I live in Connecticut. I reasonably suspect that many of the millions of U.S. citizens who live in the Southwest as neighbors or near-neighbors to Mexico and in states with significant Mexican-American populations have some knowledge of the quality, availability, and cost of medical care on the other side of the Rio Grande River. For another thing, I could not help but notice during my research for this book that a high number of the anecdotal horror stories about having cosmetic surgery abroad involve surgery performed in Mexico.

You might say that one could expect this. After all, the media in the Southwest pays attention to Mexico for news that affects those who live along the border. Also, I've already noted that far more U.S. citizens go to Mexico for inexpensive cosmetic surgery and other medical care than to any other country. The more who go, the greater the likelihood of bad experiences, even if the word is spread anecdotally.

But the number of negative stories I uncovered seemed somehow disproportionate to other countries and gave credence to the notion that Mexico was somehow a chancier destination than others. I was surprised (and frustrated) at the lack of information online that might refute the bad first impression. It is not a good sign, I thought, that I could find out more online about medical tourism in Costa Rica in an evening than I could about Mexico in a month. I put Mexico aside, more than once.

THE BAD (AND GOOD) PRESS

In February 2005, the *San Antonio Express-News* published a collection of stories and information about south-of-the-border cosmetic surgery under the headline "Beauty on the Cheap: New Body, What Price?" Reporter Lisa Marie Gómez and photojournalist Nicole Fruge spent two months on the stories. The Associated Press and MSNBC quickly picked up the reporting. Gómez's tale contained elements of horror, certainly, and what emerged was a harsh portrait of some of the dangers and pos-sible horrendous consequences of going to Mexico for cosmetic surgery. But this was not at all a piece of hit-and-run journalism, nor was it pre-sented all that sensationally, as so-called "horror stories" go. The report-ing detailed how a trip south of the border for cosmetic surgery could go terribly wrong. But the piece also said that there are good plastic surgeons in Mexico who have concerns about quality, and it told people what to look out for and how to have a better chance at a successful surgical outcome.

The story was passed around on Internet cosmetic surgery abroad forums and is still a must-read for anyone planning to go to Mexico—or anywhere else—for cosmetic surgery. The story is relatively easy to find on the Internet. (Search www.mysanantonio.com for "Special Reports".)

Gómez told me in an e-mail that she found most of her expert sources for "Beauty on the Cheap" when she attended a plastic surgery confer-ence in Canada. "Some of the best docs from Mexico were there to teach the American doctors a thing or two about face-lifts," she said. She wasn't being facetious; at international conferences and training seminars, tal-ent and experience, not nationality, are first considerations as to who is selected to present or teach.

Even working in such close proximity to Mexico, she said she found it difficult to research the story. "The hardest part about going to Mexico is finding information about the clinics and the doctors," she told me. "If it weren't for the fact that I was a reporter investigating this topic, they [Mexican officials and sources] would have shut me out." I didn't feel so bad about having had similar trouble from a greater distance.

After the story ran, Gómez and Tolbert Wilkinson, M.D., a prominent San Antonio cosmetic surgeon, hosted an online chat about the story. I couldn't resist getting in on the chat and asking a question slanted more toward the possibilities of traveling to Mexico for surgery:

The story certainly made it clear that going to Mexico for cosmetic surgery can be hazardous to one's health. A cautionary tale. However—and I address my question to Dr. Wilkinson as well— do you doubt that there are—in Mexico and other countries—highly qualified cosmetic surgeons working in facilities that are beyond reproach, and that patients who do their homework can save money and have a great experience?

Gómez answered first. "Through my research I found there are great physicians in Mexico and along the border," she replied. "The best way to find out if they are qualified is to ask for their credentials and check to see if they are board certified." She also recommended checking with people who have had surgery from them. "The point is—do your homework and double check it. It's hard to figure out if the clinics are accredited. Make them show you proof of their accreditation. Even then, check out the facility, if you can, before you have surgery. Also, listen to your gut. A lot of the patients I talked to said their instincts told them not to have surgery at a particular clinic, and did it anyway. They later regretted it."

I expected that Dr. Wilkinson would perhaps be a little harsher. A surgeon with 30 years experience, he told Gómez that he has had dozens of patients who came to him for repairs after bad surgery in Mexico. But he was careful to draw a distinction between good Mexican surgeons and bad ones. "Just because a doctor is certified does not necessarily mean he or she is qualified," he told me. He went on to say that "Some of the best plastic surgeons in the world are in Guadalajara and Mexico City." But he cautioned about the border doctors, who may not be trained plastic surgeons. "The people on the border don't give a damn," he told the *Express-News*. "They're giving all the excellent, properly trained Mexican surgeons a bad name."

> "Just because a doctor is certified does not necessarily mean he or she is qualified."

PROCEED—BUT WITH CAUTION

The message was loud and clear: People interested in inexpensive cosmetic surgery should be extremely careful when choosing a surgeon and a facility, and there seem to be more suspect doctors and sub-par facilities in the border towns of Mexico than elsewhere. Once again, however, it's unreasonable and unfair to tar all, or even most, of the medical professionals in a geographic area with the same brush. There are good doctors and bad doctors everywhere, and there are many well-qualified, board-certified cosmetic surgeons working in Mexico, catering to patients from the United States and charging far less than their U.S. peers. That includes the border towns.

> There seem to be more suspect doctors and more sub-par facilities in the border towns of Mexico than anywhere else.

The vast majority of the thousands of people who go to Mexico from the United States for more affordable surgery, medical care, or dental work presumably are not desperate or foolish. They generally do their homework, check credentials, get referrals, and plan ahead. There are, after all, more than 900 board-certified plastic and cosmetic surgeons working in Mexico, according to the Mexican Association of Plastic, Aesthetic and Reconstructive Surgery. The association has an extensive English-language Web site at: **www.plasticsurgery.org.mx.**

Jaime Caloca Jr., M.D., is one of about 30 board-certified Mexican cosmetic surgeons open for business just in Tijuana. Caloca and his father have been in practice together for 17 years. Their offices and recently remodeled surgical suite are in the modern "Rio Zone" in Tijuana, about 20 miles south of San Diego. He is just one of a number of Mexican surgeons with whom I corresponded over a period of months in 2005, but his comments were the most broadly representative. He could not estimate the number of U.S. patients who go to Mexico annually (a number I have put at 40,000 or so), but guessed that 80 percent of those who do, go to the border towns and cities, as opposed to Mexico City or resort areas.

Dr. Caloca defended the reputable surgeons who practice along the border, while acknowledging that problems exist. Reputable surgeons should work together across borders, he argued.

"I am very much aware of U.S. individuals and associations and their pressures to discredit any and all plastic surgeons outside of the United States. The main error is that they generalize," Dr. Caloca said. "There may be unprepared and unethical physicians (and even persons who claim to be physicians but are not) in any country. I have seen patients who fall into the hands of these charlatans in both the United States and in Mexico and have horrible results. We should all be opposing the charlatans together...both United States and Mexican surgeons must unite in informing patients on how to choose a qualified plastic surgeon, whether it be in the United States, Mexico, or anywhere else in the world."

Dr. Caloca was among the several surgeons I spoke to who do not think that Mexican surgeons—or any cosmetic surgeons abroad—are taking business away from their peers in the United States. Instead, he argued, they are providing services for those who cannot afford U.S. prices.

"I sincerely think that we do not subtract patients from U.S. plastic surgery practices, since most of our patients would not be able to get services in the United States anyway due to the high costs," he said. "I can tell you as a fact that most U.S. patients that come to me from my Web site would have had their surgeries in the United States if they had the economic means to do so. These patients would not have even searched away from their country if the cost was not so ridiculously high.

"On the other hand, there is the patient—and I have had many—that does have the money to get plastic surgery in Beverly Hills or wherever, but prefers to come to me because their best friend or their mother or their friend had surgery with us and are happy with their results."

U.S. and Mexican board-certified surgeons actually do meet monthly. Dr. Caloca said the San Diego Plastic Surgery Society meetings are "informal, but productive."

INSIDE MEXICO

One might think that U.S. citizens would generally have fewer misconceptions about Mexico than other countries. The **United States and Mexico share a 2,000-mile border**, a lengthy (and occasionally bloody) history, and have extensively blended cultures in much of the American Southwest. An average of more than 40,000 people from the United States visit Mexico every day. The farther one gets from the border, though, the less likely one is to know much about Mexico beyond the national news, which is dominated by immigration and trade issues. When Mexico sent aid to New Orleans after Hurricane Katrina devastated the city, it prompted jokes on television. Bill Maher, host of *Real Time* on HBO, got laughs by saying something along the lines of "You know the U.S. is in trouble when we're getting emergency food and clean drinking water from Mexico."

Old stereotypes die hard.

Old stereotypes die hard. Mexico has substantially improved its infrastructure in the last 20 years and experts insist the tap water in most areas is safe. Medical care is generally of high quality in urban areas, though, as everywhere else, one has to research, check references, do one's homework.

The Language Barrier

The national language is, of course, **Spanish. English is spoken widely but by no means universally. Doctors, surgeons, and dentists who cater to U.S. patients generally speak English.**

Geography

Everyone in the United States knows where Mexico is, but many do not have a good conception of how big and diverse a country it is. **Mexico is nearly three times the size of Texas** and has a population of more than 100 million people.

More than 24 million people live in and around **Mexico City, making it the most populous metropolitan area in the world.** At more than 7,500 feet above sea level, it is also one of the highest. The six largest border towns are Ciudad Juárez, Tijuana, Mexicali, Matamoros, Reynosa, and Nuevo Laredo. Each, in combination with its "sister city"—the neighboring U.S. city right across the border—has a population of more than 500,000. Far from being the "border towns" that many U.S. residents farther north might imagine, these are significant metropolitan areas, among the fastest growing in the hemisphere, as this chart shows:

Metropolitan Area	Population (2000)	Population (1990)	Change
San Diego (CA)/ Tijuana	4,065,359	3,245,397	25.3%
El Paso (TX)/ Ciudad Juárez	1,930,756	1,389,709	38.9%
Rio Bravo (TX)/ Reynosa	1,073,720	760,221	41.2%
Imperial County (CA)/ Mexicali	913,787	711,241	28.5%
Brownsville (TX)/ Matamoros	752,460	563,413	33.6%
Laredo (TX)/ Nuevo Laredo	509,451	352,807	44.4%

(Source: www.demographia.com)

These metro areas also have the problems of most rapidly growing urban areas, including pollution, traffic, and crime—but they have attracted some of the leading cosmetic surgeons and dentists in Mexico because of their proximity to the large and relatively affluent market in the United States. As doctors on both sides of the border point out, they have also attracted perhaps more than their share of charlatans, frauds, and incompetents.

Many Mexican plastic surgeons also are in practice in the country's beach resort areas, catering to an international clientele. Mexico City, Guadalajara, and major tourist areas are easily accessible via direct flight from most U.S. cities.

U.S. patients who live near the border generally can recuperate at home. Those who travel farther can elect surgery south of the border and recovery on the U.S. side. Reputable, board-certified surgeons generally work in their own modern facilities or in modern private hospitals. But the northern part of the country is also "littered" with "backward operations run by physicians of questionable credentials," according to the *San Antonio Express-News*. Here, as elsewhere, shopping for cosmetic surgery or dentistry on price alone is absurd and asking for trouble.

Infrastructure

As Dr. Caloca noted, perhaps half of Mexico's 900 or so cosmetic surgeons have at least some patients from abroad. Those who are more experienced with caring for international patients often work in conjunction with patient referral services, "recovery haciendas," resorts, or other local accommodations so that they are able to offer package deals. Prospective patients should ask surgeons about their recommended accommodations.

Marketing

Many Mexican surgeons have their own English-language Web sites, though not nearly as many as one might expect, especially if you compare them to the number of Costa Rican sites. Part of the reason may well go back, again, to proximity, Mexico's No. 1 advantage in medical tourism. Mexican surgeons in the border towns are, effectively, already working in U.S. metropolitan areas. They can advertise by more traditional means and it is not difficult for them to market their services in person in the United States. Similarly, surgeons in resort/beach areas in Mexico locate there because of the huge number of tourists, and prices are generally higher.

HOW TO FIND A SURGEON

Search the Web, browse the forums and support groups, learn from the experiences of others—but start with **the Mexican Association of Plastic,**

Aesthetic and Reconstructive Surgery's Web site, mentioned earlier in this chapter (www.platicsurgery.org.mx). Though board certification is not a guarantee of a surgeon's talent, lack of certification makes for a huge question mark. The site has a full directory of member surgeons and contact information.

THE COUNTRY

For U.S. citizens, there are **three Mexicos**. There is the **Mexico of the border cities**, generally friendly towards tourists, more prosperous, accessible, and newer than much of the rest of the country. The border zone by law extends 20 kilometers (about 12 miles) into Mexico. U.S. residents can enter and stay for up to 72 hours with just a valid proof of citizenship (U.S. passport preferred).

You can walk, take public transportation, or drive into a border area. If you intend to undergo surgery during your stay, presumably you will go by car. You'll need Mexican auto insurance, obtainable in advance or at the border; Mexico generally does not recognize U.S. insurance as valid.

Then there is the **Mexico beyond the border zones**. You'll need a tourist card, also known as an FM-T. If you wish to drive or be driven, you'll need a temporary importation permit for the vehicle. Beyond that, if you are not accustomed to traveling through Mexico by private car, you may want to think twice about doing so for the first time as a medical tourist. Some destinations and roads are considered unsafe for motorists for a variety of reasons. Check online travel guides (search for "Driving in Mexico"), and consult with others who have driven into the Mexican interior.

Finally, there is the Mexico that is most familiar to U.S. citizens—**the resort areas and the major interior cities**, the Mexico that is on the other end of a flight itinerary. Doctors and surgeons in these locations who are accustomed to treating patients from abroad should be able to recommend local accommodations, transportation, and personal references. If they can not, try another surgeon. And don't expect them all to be similarly inexpensive. Top international surgeons, or even just popular ones, charge more, especially in wealthy and resort areas.

CHAPTER 10

The Far East: The New "Cutting Edge" in Medical Tourism

The thing about modern medical tourism in the Far East is that it really wasn't there until what seems like just a minute ago. I hate having to say that. I like looking at the lineage of events, and would love to digress and go back to the earliest days of doctoring in China and India and the ancient techniques that are still in use, and still revered, today. Or at least dwell for a while on the current King of Thailand's father, who graduated from both Harvard Medical School and the Harvard School of Public Health. (His Majesty King Bhumipol Adulyadej was born on December 5, 1927 at Mount Auburn Hospital in Cambridge, Massachusetts.)

But for all practical purposes, modern medical tourism in Asia has its roots no further back than about 1997, when Bumrungrad Hospital in Bangkok, Thailand opened a new, ultra-modern 554-bed facility. It seemed a chancy venture to some at the time. The Asian economy was in the throes of a major currency crisis and there was no certainty that Bumrungrad, originally a 200-bed hospital built in 1980, would be successful on a large scale. Nor was Bumrungrad the only hospital modernizing and looking abroad for patients. But the guiding philosophy seemed to be "build it and they will come." Bumrungrad targeted foreign patients with an aggressive marketing strategy.

They came. By 2002, Bumrungrad had welcomed 250,000 patients from outside Thailand. In 2004, it was named the "Best Small Cap Company" by the Singapore-based magazine *Asiamoney*, which called the hospital "a remarkable success story." In accepting the award, Bumrungrad Group CEO Curtis J. Schroeder said: "Bumrungrad has made a remarkable recovery from the dark days of the Asian economic crisis through an effective restructuring and has emerged as the dominant regional player in the Southeast Asian health-care market for cost-effective international medical care."

Then, in April 2005, CBS and *60 Minutes* showed up in Thailand and at Apollo Hospitals in India. Like I said, it all happened in about a minute—suddenly the American media was paying attention. In Thailand, in India, in Malaysia—once the business opportunity for U.S. patients was identified, corporations went after it. They built hospitals to U.S. standards, and staffed them with U.S.-trained doctors and surgeons. India has gone after the medical services business with

> Hospitals are built to U.S. standards and staffed by U.S.-trained doctors and surgeons.

the same vigor it has shown in gaining market share in, say, software development and customer service call centers.

THAILAND—CAPITAL OF MEDICAL TOURISM

Thailand is, at least for now, the capital of the medical tourism world. **Bumrungrad Hospital** is its palace and Curtis Schroeder is its king. Of the 350,000 international patients treated at the hospital in 2004, 50,000 were from the United States. When Bumrungrad was featured on *60 Minutes*, more than 3,000 patient inquiries from the United States poured in the next day. The story showed the hospital in such an extraordinarily favorable light that the hospital linked its main hospital Web page **(www.bumrungrad.com)** to the CBS show's Web site. The patient statements sound as though they could have been written by the hospital's marketing department, but they weren't. U.S. patients were not only happy with saving approximately 80 percent on their health care costs; they also weren't shy about saying that the care they received was not just as good as, but better than what they would have expected in the United States.

"I found it so strange in Thailand, because they were all registered nurses. Being in a hospital in the United States, we see all kinds of orderlies, all kinds of aides, maybe one R.N. on duty on the whole floor of the hospital," said Byron Bonnewell of Louisiana, who had quintuple bypass surgery at Bumrungrad for $12,000 instead of the $100,000 it would have cost him in the United States. "In Thailand, I bet I had eight R.N.s just on my section of the floor alone. First-class care."

Bumrungrad: Five-Star Accommodations

Ruben Toral, Bumrungrad's director of international programs, sums it up with some pride. "We offer a complete package—very high medical and service standards, a five-star facility and very competitive prices. Where else can you walk in without an appointment, see a board-certified specialist in under 15 minutes, pay U.S. $15 for the consultation, and have a Starbucks cappuccino on your way out? That's really quite unique."

Bumrungrad's claim of five-star status isn't idle hype for either inpatient or outpatient accommodations. A single deluxe room in the hospital with personal VCR, private marble bathroom, refrigerator, microwave, dishes, glasses, and a granite dining table costs less than $100 a night. Non-private inpatient rooms are about $25. At the top of the scale, the royal suite with a guestroom runs about $365 a night. For recovering outpatients and their families or guests, Bumrungrad has 74 attached residence apartments and suites; a studio apartment is less than $30 a night, and a VIP suite is less than $90.

There are more than 700 doctors and surgeons affiliated with Bumrungrad, many of them trained and/or board certified in the United States. Most speak English. The hospital itself was the first in Asia to formally meet U.S. JCAHO standards.

There is nothing not to like about Bumrungrad for patients from the United States, other than the 18-to-24-hour travel time. Do some really rigorous research on the Internet and you will find a few patients who were not entirely happy, for various reasons, but not very many. Whatever medical tourism will mean for the future of health care in the United States in terms of costs and access to care, Bumrungrad's success will be, in some part, a measure of it.

A single deluxe hospital room with personal VCR, private marble bath, refrigerator, dishes, glasses, and a granite dining table costs less than $100 a night.

Bumrungrad has made a point of presenting itself to the world as a full-service, state-of-the-art international hospital, rather than pushing any particular specialty.

Certainly, that patients from the United States go there for quintuple heart bypass surgery somehow bestows more instant credibility than that they go there for liposuction. Yet, even at Bumrungrad, one of the main lures for prospective visitors from the United States is plastic or cosmetic surgery—about 20 percent or 10,000 of the 50,000 or so Americans who go there annually. The Bumrungrad Web site's link "Find a Doctor" features 18 English-speaking, board-certified cosmetic and plastic surgeons working at the hospital at last count. A full range of cosmetic surgery "all-inclusive" packages are advertised.

Other Quality Hospitals

Bumrungrad is certainly the best publicized medical tourism destination in Thailand, and attracts roughly 50 percent of all medical tourists visiting the country. But those who want to comparison shop have plenty of options. Among the other leading hospitals that cater to international patients is **Yanhee General Hospital (www.yanhee.net)**, a 400-bed full-service modern facility in Bangkok with a particularly good reputation for cosmetic surgery. The Tourism Authority of Thailand **(www.tourismthailand.com)** recognizes medical tourism as a "product," and maintains a list of hospitals with Web site and contact information.

Bangkok Hospital (www.bangkokhospital.com), the flagship of the **Dusit Medical Group**, treated roughly 100,000 patients from abroad in 2005 in its 14 hospitals throughout the country. Some of Bangkok Hospital's marketing material makes veiled reference to the Bumrungrad glitziness, which has seemingly set the bar for private hospitals throughout Asia:

Many Thai, Singaporean, and Indian hospitals have developed excellent PR services and "flashy looks" to cater to their foreign clients. There are people who know about it and pay inquisitive attention to these non-medical matters. Some get carried away by the big restaurants, coffee shops, apartment rooms, etc. and consider these services as the standard bearer of medical care in that hospital. The local people often do not care about these matters. They know the situation well and devote

attention almost exclusively to the medical matters. There are some
hospitals that have few local patients but a large number of foreigners.
One should ask why the locals don't go there for treatment if it is a
good hospital.

It's a competitive business. Both **Bumrungrad** and the **Dusit Medical
Group** are investing millions of dollars in new facilities in Thailand and
overseas. Dusit Medical Group is investing in a hospital in **southern
China**. Bumrungrad is managing new private hospitals in **Bangladesh**
and **Myanmar**, and in 2005 acquired a 39 percent stake in Manila's **Asian
Hospital** in the **Philippines**. It also is taking a 49 percent share in a
$40 million health care complex in **Dubai** in the United Arab Emirates,
which is intended to become a medical hub for the Middle East and
North Africa. "At a certain point, people aren't going to come here to
Bumrungrad in Thailand," Toral has said. "They will want different
options, and that's what we're creating."

The Language Barrier
Thai is the official language, though **English is spoken widely** in the
tourism industry and certainly by doctors, surgeons, and front-line staff
of the major hospitals that compete for medical tourism business.
English is taught as a second language in Thai schools.

Geography
Thailand is in **Southeast Asia**, bordered by Malaysia to the south and
additionally enclosed by Burma, Laos, and Cambodia, with a lengthy
coastline along the Gulf of Thailand. The country is about twice the size
of Wyoming and has a population of about 66 million people.

    Bangkok, a city with a metropolitan population of 9 million, is the most
common destination by far for medical tourists, though the island of **Phuket**
(pronounced, roughly, "poo-get") is becoming a destination in its own right.
But there is no getting around the fact that Thailand is a long way away
from the United States and Western Europe. For rough planning and comparison purposes, budget about $1,000 for airfare and then shop around.

Infrastructure

Thailand has modern hospitals that were built with the care of medical tourists in mind. Health tourism is also big in Thailand, with **renowned luxury spas, and recovery and wellness retreats and resorts.** A prospective patient from abroad can make complete arrangements through a hospital, work through one of numerous patient service companies based in Thailand, book through a medical tourism company based in the United States, or mix and match.

Marketing

Medical care in Thailand is easy to research. Even a cursory search of the Internet will turn up a wealth of information, in addition to the major hospital sites mentioned above. There is not, as yet, as much in the way of Internet patient-support forums and message boards as there are for South and Central American destination countries.

Thailand has become a leading destination for patients **seeking gender reassignment surgery**, though the major hospitals generally do not specifically mention the surgery on their Web sites. Information about doctors who perform the surgery is easy to find, however, as are patient reviews and forums for the transgendered who have had surgery overseas.

How to Find a Surgeon

The **Society of Plastic and Reconstructive Surgeons of Thailand** maintains a Web site with both Thai- and English-language versions at: **www.plasticsurgery.or.th.** The site's "Find Plastic Surgeon" page warns that any doctor in Thailand with a license to practice medicine can practice cosmetic surgery, as is the case in the United States and other countries. Interestingly, it makes a point of saying that "some of the best cosmetic surgeons in Thailand rarely advertise," though quite a number of cosmetic surgeons in Thailand do have their own Web sites. In the absence of any other information, however, the wisest course seems to be to inquire directly through the Web sites of the major international hospitals or go through a medical tourism company that can offer references.

Getting Around the Country

Thailand has been a **constitutional monarchy** since 1932 and a **close ally of the United States** since after World War II. **Bangkok** is a modern, vibrant city and its airport is a key point for international travelers. The country's dependence on agriculture has lessened substantially in the past 20 years, but it still exports more rice than any other nation in the world. The economy is one of the fastest growing in the world. Services and infrastructure in Bangkok are on a par with any major international city. A passport is required for entry into the country, but there is no visa requirement for visitors staying less than 30 days.

Parts of the **western coast** are still recovering from the effects of the tsunami that devasted the region in December 2004, but most tourist areas reopened within days or weeks of the disaster. Bangkok was unaffected by the tsunami.

The U.S. Department of State notes that the threat of crime in Bangkok is lower than it is in most cities in the United States but visitors should exercise the same caution they would in any urban area.

There are certain misconceptions that people in the United States may have about the country formerly known as Siam. It is worth noting that the story of "Anna and the King," celebrated in the classic Broadway musical "The King and I" and made several times into popular movies, is regarded in Thailand, with reason, as gross fiction and a grave insult to Thai culture, history, and the institution of the monarchy. The movie versions of the story are banned in the country. As with anywhere else, it is a good idea for visitors to familiarize themselves at least somewhat with the culture before traveling. The Thai people are generally warm and welcoming to tourists, particularly those from the United States.

INDIA: EXPECTING TO LEAD THE WAY

Looming both over and yet somehow slightly behind Thailand in the development of medical tourism is **India**, where very big things are expected. Perhaps because of India's notable successes in garnering a significant share of the U.S. market for outsourced services, the country is perceived by some experts as poised to dominate as a world supplier of health care, and for good reasons. **The Apollo Hospitals Group (www.apollohospitals.com)** was co-featured with Bumrungrad Hospital on *60 Minutes* and written about approvingly in the *Wall Street Journal*.

India seems to have everything going for it—new hospitals, rapidly improving urban infrastructure, outstanding and experienced doctors and surgeons, the makings of a general tourism boom, the will and dynamism of one of the world's fastest-growing economies, and, just as important, prices for medical care even lower than those in Thailand. "It makes sense to establish India as sort of a world destination for health care," Anjali Kapoor Bissell, director of Apollo's International Patient Office, told *60 Minutes*.

> India has everything going for it—new hospitals, outstanding doctors, and prices even lower than those found in Thailand.

Well, yes, it does. But still, despite the investments, despite the hype, Thailand is still the leader in medical tourism in the Far East and pulling away. What's wrong? Nothing, really, other than that India, due to an unbroken string of successes in building its economy, perhaps suffers from extraordinarily high expectations. The fact is, India has never been a major world tourist destination before. Building new hospitals and offering high-quality inexpensive medical care helps put India on the map, but it has a long way to go. Roughly 14 million foreigners visited Thailand in 2004. Fewer than 4 million tourists came to India. That's a huge gap in exposure and recognition to make up.

The Economic Times of India, in a September 2005 article headlined "Are Hospitals Ready for Medical Tourism?" forthrightly noted that perhaps the country has a way to go in attracting patients from the United States and Western Europe, as opposed to just from Asia. "Initial efforts and representations from the Indian hospitals to the health-care bodies in the United Kingdom and United States to ease pressure and waiting queues in their country by diverting patients to India hasn't yielded encouraging results. That has sent most industry players to put best possible infrastructure and services as a bait," the *Times* reported, quoting a senior executive with a Chennai-based private hospital chain.

Despite glowing reports from abroad, India's medical tourism business was viewed in the article as an underachiever, even though growth has been estimated at 10-15 percent annually.

The government's response was to set up a task force to suggest ways to better promote India as a health-care destination. It also moved toward passing laws to standardize quality in health-care facilities and to make it easier for medical tourists to enter the country. And the **Indian Tourism Ministry** vowed to target 10 to 15 tourist areas in the country for rapid modernization. A month later the **Ministries of Health and Tourism** announced that it would jointly sponsor a Web site for medical tourism. As of this writing, the site had not been launched.

None of this means that India is not already an excellent option as a medical tourist destination, or that it will not realize its potential in time. The Apollo Group hospitals, in particular, are succeeding in drawing patients from the United States and Europe who are happy with both the quality of care and the prices in India. But this is not a market that India is likely to dominate, or even lead, in the near future.

U.S. Affiliates

Though the **Apollo Hospitals Group** is not the beginning and the end of medical tourism in India, the company is by far the **largest private health-care provider in the country** and has taken the lead in developing the medical tourism business. The company's hospitals are modern, with the latest technology and equipment; its patient accommodations are luxurious and inexpensive. Those are the standards for competing in the Far East. Seventy percent of Apollo's doctors and surgeons have trained, studied, or worked in institutions and hospitals in the West. The company has affiliations with **Royal College of Surgeons of Edinburgh; New**

> 70 percent of Apollo's doctors and surgeons have trained, studied, or worked in the West.

York Hospital / Cornell Medical Center; Galvin Heart Center in
Evanston, Illinois; Pomona Valley Hospital Medical Center, California;
Sloan-Kettering Institute, New York; and the American Heart
Association, among others, for training and staff development.

Apollo Hospitals can directly handle all aspects of a prospective
patient's trip, including all travel arrangements, coordination of doctor's
appointments, accommodations for relatives and attendants, cuisine
options, interpreters, and arrangements for post-operative recuperation
at a leading resort.

Indian Doctors, U.S. Trained

In the United States one in 20 doctors is Indian or Indian-American. The
best and brightest in India have long gravitated to the West for medical
and science education and training. More and more, however, there are
opportunities for them to return and work in their home country, in facilities comparable to those in which they trained. In growing numbers, the
patients from the United States follow. There is no common major procedure or surgery that one can not have done in India, and there are several that are done nowhere else—hip resurfacing, as opposed to hip replacement, is one example. Hip resurfacing is not yet approved in the United States; the technique was developed in India, and that is one procedure that attracts patients to India. Of course, patients travel to India for inexpensive cosmetic surgery, as well.

> There are no procedures that can not be done in India, and there are several that can not be done anywhere else.

The Language Barrier

Hindi is the national language but English is, in effect, an associate
national language and more important than Hindi for national, political,
and business communication.

Geography
India is the **largest country on what is often referred to as the South Asian subcontinent**; it is about **one-third the size of the United States** and pokes into the Indian Ocean between the Arabian Sea and the Bay of Bengal. The country is bordered to the north by Nepal, China, and Pakistan. Bangladesh, to the northeast, is almost surrounded by India; Burma is to the east. The **population is about 1.1 billion**.

Mumbai (formerly Bombay), Delhi, Calcutta, Bangalore, Chennai (Madras), Ahmedabad, and **Hyderabad** are the largest cities. India has at least a little of everything, geographically, in a country that ranges from the tropics to the Himalayan peaks.

For rough planning purposes, budget $1,200 to $1,500 for airfare from the United States. When shopping for flights, check for possible bargains that combine deals on fares from the United States to Great Britain with budget fares from Great Britain to India.

Infrastructure
India is a nation undergoing an economic transformation at a speed and scale without precedent, other than in China. A vast middle class has emerged. Still, most of the population lives in rural areas and in relative poverty. Tourists may find the squalor of the cities alarming, but the hospitals and accommodations are first class.

Marketing
It is easy to find news on the Internet about medical tourism in India and there are major medical tourism companies with significant resources online. **Medical Tourism India (www.indiamedicaltourism.net)** is one example, but there are dozens of them. The **Ministry of Tourism (www.tourisminindia.com)** has some splendid information about the country, but as of this writing there is nothing "official" noted about medical tourism—though the ministry does take advertisements on the site, and the Jaipur Dental Hospital has been a sponsor, promising savings of 90 percent compared to the United States. I have little doubt that online resources for medical tourism in India will increase substantially in the future.

How to Find a Surgeon

There is no comprehensive Web site for the Association of Plastic Surgeons of India. Medical tourists interested in cosmetic surgery are probably best off working through a medical-tourism company, or directly through one of the major hospitals—most likely one of those owned or run by the Apollo Group. Prospective patients for all other procedures should probably start at the Apollo Web site, though there are a few other private hospital companies with fine reputations, such as **Escorts Heart Institute and Research Center (www.ehirc.com)** in New Delhi. The institute is recognized as a leader in cardiac surgery, interventional cardiology, pediatric surgery, and cardiac diagnostics, and specializes in offering surgery to high-risk patients. It bills itself as unique in offering "a fully developed program of monitored exercise, yoga, and meditation for lifestyle and stress management."

The prices, again, are less than a quarter of what would typically be charged in the United States, perhaps even closer to a tenth for major procedures.

The Country

Most Westerners have a dichotomous view of India. Lingering is the perception that the country is overpopulated, impoverished, and unhealthy—an enormous and troubled world in need of a thousand Mother Teresas. Superimposed over that mental image, however, is that of an emerging India, one which produces doctors, scientists, and engineers at a pace unmatched other than in China; one which is a juggernaut of technical services, favored by U.S. companies for outsourcing jobs and significant business functions. Both Indias are real.

Medical tourism, of course, is part of the emerging India, and prospective patients should concentrate on that. While this is a gross oversimplification, it is a useful one for a prospective medical tourist. India merits serious consideration as a destination, particularly for those in the United States who are uninsured or underinsured but require expensive surgery or treatment. For lesser surgery and for cosmetic surgery, India is also an option, particularly (and obviously) for those who have always wanted to go there. India is working on providing more compelling reasons for more people to want to visit.

A valid passport and visa is required for entry. **The Indian Embassy in Washington, D.C.** has an extensive Web site with information for travelers at: **www.indianembassy.org.**

MALAYSIA: SILICONE VALLEY OF SOUTHEAST ASIA

While Thailand and India have garnered most of the media attention in the United States as medical tourism destinations in Asia, **Malaysia** has simultaneously worked to raise its profile and establish itself as a viable option. More than 100,000 foreigners now visit the country annually for medical treatment and surgery, according to the government. The Malaysian government is actively promoting medical tourism. When MedRetreat, a U.S. medical tourism company, sent its first cosmetic surgery patients to Malaysia in the spring of 2005, a post-trip media conference was hosted at the Malaysian Embassy in Washington, D.C.

Whereas Thailand and India have avoided putting cosmetic surgery front and center in marketing medical care, Malaysian officials have not been shy about doing so. **Penang Island,** off the Malaysian coast, has been called the Silicone Valley of Southeast Asia. It aspires to be compared to Beverly Hills, as well. Kee Phaik Cheen, Penang state tourism committee chairman, told *Agence France-Presse* in 2005 that the future of the medical industry in Penang is bright. In a memorable if slightly off-color quote, Cheen added, "As tourism chief, I am happy. You can enjoy the sun, the beach, and go home with a good set of new boobs."

> "You can enjoy the sun, the beach, and go home with a good set of new boobs."

A closer look at the available information, however, indicates that Malaysia so far is drawing most of its medical tourists from the immediate region and very few from the United States or Europe. Moreover, most of the visits are for checkups or minor health problems. The numbers tell the story even when government officials are trying to sound optimistic. In a May 2005 interview with the Middle East business Web portal **www.strategiy.com** (put the I in your strategy), Deputy Minister of Tourism Ahmad Zahid Hamidi was characteristically upbeat:

> In fact Malaysia is also fast emerging as a value-for-money destination for health and medical tourism. We have world-class health and medical facilities. In 2004 alone, a total of more than 129,318 foreign patients received medical treatment in the country, generating foreign exchange earnings of RM105 million [$27.63 million]. Malaysia's health and medical tourism are picking up because of favorable exchange rates and a wide choice of private medical centers with highly qualified medical professionals.

And that sounds great—until you divide $27.63 million by 129,318 patients and come up with an average expenditure per patient of $213.66, which does not buy a lot of cosmetic surgery even at Malaysian prices.

By later in the year, the Malaysian Minister of Health was sounding a more cautious note. "As far as medical tourism goes, the government is for it, but... it is the private sector which is the engine of growth for this segment," Datuk Chua Soi Lek, M.D., told the *Business Times* of Malaysia, indicating that the medical tourism sector was not going to reach revenue projections. "The ministry only provides the infrastructure. As for the promotion, it is up to them [private sector]."

Dr. Chua said private hospitals were not providing the ministry with requested data about foreign patients." We do not have a clear picture," he said, adding that Malaysian hospitals should also be looking at providing high-end treatment as opposed to just health screening, dental procedures or breast implants.

As with India, just because medical tourism isn't drawing as many patients from the West as Malaysian officials had hoped—in other words, not as many as Thailand—does not mean that there is anything wrong with the health care. The media conference at the Malaysian Embassy in April 2005 was a small showcase for the country and what it has to offer, which is not notably different than what one can find in Bangkok.

Two patients from the United States, one of them a registered nurse, spoke at the press conference about their wonderful experience in going to Malaysia for cosmetic surgery. They were reassured before they went abroad that their surgeon, Danny Oh, M.D., had 27 years of experience and is a member of the American Society of Plastic Surgeons. Their hospital, Penang Adventist, was ultramodern; their outpatient accommodations, five-star; the total price for surgery and two weeks abroad was less than they would have paid for surgery at home. MedRetreat handled the arrangements.

In Malaysia, a MedRetreat partner, Beautiful Holidays, shepherded the patients from arrival to departure. The trip was perfect. That it was documented every step of the way for public relations purposes did not detract from the patients' satisfaction with the results, or make it anything other than what anyone else could expect if they did the same thing.

Somehow, though, it just wasn't news. The media conference was sparsely attended. There can be a lot of reasons why this happens. Luck and timing have a lot to do with it. My own speculation is at that precise moment, the Malaysians and MedRetreat were just a little too late. By April 2005, the media knew the story, had done that. In fact, I had just about given up on trying to get magazine assignments to do that kind of reporting. The story was morphing into "lots of people are doing this." Two weeks later, *60 Minutes* featured Bumrungrad and India. Malaysia remained...undiscovered.

The Language Barrier

Bahasa Malaysia is the official language but **English is widely spoken—** the region was under the political and economic control of Great Britain from the 18th century until independence in the 1950s and the British influence remains apparent.

Geography

The Federation of Malaysia is **comprised mostly of the peninsula in Southeast Asia it shares with Thailand to the north, plus the northern**

third of the island of Borneo. The country's population is about 26 million people.

The major international city is **Kuala Lumpur**, population 1.5 million, home of the Petronas Towers, among the world's tallest buildings. **Putrajaya**, a planned city founded in 1995, is the official seat of government. As with other Asian destinations, it is a long way from home for U.S. travelers. Figure on 18-to-24 hours of travel time and, for rough planning purposes, budget $1,000 for airfare.

Infrastructure

The **urban areas of Malaysia are as modern** as those of anywhere else in the world, if not more so. The private hospitals meet international standards and many of the doctors and surgeons trained and/or have worked in the United States and Europe.

Malaysia was spared a direct hit by the Asian tsunami of December 2004, and its tourism industry was only minimally affected for a short period.

Marketing

If there were a first prize for the best Web site devoted to the medical tourism resources of a particular country, the **Association of Private Hospitals of Malaysia (APHM, www.hospitals-malaysia.org)** would win hands down. Although only about 35 hospitals and medical facilities in Malaysia out of more than 200 are actively marketing medical tourism, at least to the extent of participating in the Web site, the APHM site provides a great drive-by on what Malaysia has to offer. It provides detailed snapshots and Web addresses for all of the private hospitals in the country that are courting medical tourists. All of the hospitals listed have extensive English-language Web sites.

A number of medical tourism companies include or even specialize in Malaysia as a destination. Two with which I've become familiar offer excellent Web sites and references. The aforementioned **Beautiful Holidays (www.beautiful-holidays.com)** is one; another is **Gorgeous Getaways (www.gorgeousgetaways.com)**. Both offer cosmetic surgery travel packages.

However, you will not find a lot on the Internet about individual doctors or surgeons practicing in Malaysia because advertising of medical services is strictly regulated. The APHM site, though, more than makes up in quality what is missing in quantity, and medical tourism company sites fill in the blanks.

Malaysia is in the process of rather publicly branding itself as a tourist destination, an effort that will surely boost the profile of medical tourism. The focus remains more on attracting tourists from the Middle East and Europe than on the United States, however.

How to Find a Surgeon

Among other Web sites, the **Academy of Medicine of Malaysia (www.acadmed.org.my)** and the **Malaysian Association of Specialists in Private Medical Practice (www.aspmp.org)** provide searchable member directories listing more than 1,500 physicians and surgeons, although some of the better-known ones are not in it. In the absence of a specific referral, most prospective patients who are interested in cosmetic surgery or other medical care in Malaysia are best off investigating either directly through one of the private hospitals or in using the services of a medical tourism company.

Prices for medical services fall in a range established by agreement among the private hospitals and are competitive within the region (specifically and pointedly, no doubt, with those in neighboring Thailand), and are generally less than a quarter of what would typically be charged for the same services in the United States.

THE COUNTRY

Malaysia is a **constitutional democracy** and an economic success story. It is also a complex society, with Malay, Chinese, Indian, and indigenous people maintaining and mixing cultures. Medical tourism aside, Malaysia is a popular destination for its modern cities, beautiful beaches, eco-tourism, and the hospitality and genuine friendliness of its people.

A passport is required but no visa is necessary for stays of less than 90

(continued on page 184)

RATES FOR MAJOR PROCEDURES IN MALAYSIA

The Malaysian Ministry of Tourism and the Association of Private Hospitals of Malaysia (APHM) have worked in tandem to promote medical tourism in the country. The APHM has established "price bands," ranges of prices for various common procedures, for all its member hospitals, making it easier for prospective patients to evaluate Malaysia as a possible destination. The full list is available at the APHM Web site. The price ranges in this chart are examples of costs for common major surgery and cosmetic surgery procedures as of January 2006.

These figures were translated from the Malaysian currency (the Ringgit) using an exchange rate of .266 U.S. Dollars/1 Ringgit and should be used as indicators only. Actual pricing will be determined at the point of care. In the absence of complications, they would generally be within the range listed.

Procedure	Lowest Cost (U.S. Dollars)	Highest Cost	Included Services
CARDIOLOGY			
Coronary artery bypass graft	$6,630	$9,285	• 2-3 days ICU stay • Not more than 7-day stay • Inclusive of consultation charges, and cardiologist and anesthetist fees
Angioplasty (actual price depends on number of balloons/stents used)	$3,979	$5,836	• 1-day stay • Inclusive of cardiologist, procedure, and equipment charges
OPHTHALMOLOGY			
Cataract surgery	$716	$1,326	Exclusive of overnight stay

Procedure	Lowest Cost (U.S. Dollars)	Highest Cost	Included Services
ORTHOPEDIC			
Total knee replacement	$3,979	$4,775	• 5-day stay in hospital room (inclusive of meals) • Inclusive of orthopedic and anesthetist charges • Surgery charges and implant
Hip replacement	$3,979	$5,305	• 5-day hospital stay (inclusive of meals) • Includes consultation
PLASTIC SURGERY			
Double eyelid/ eyebag	$530	$663	Exclusive of overnight stay
Face and neck lift	$1,857	$2,653	Inclusive of 2-day stay
Breast augmentation	$2,122	$2,653	Exclusive of overnight stay
Breast reduction/lift	$1,857	$2,653	Inclusive of 1-day stay
Liposuction	$1,326	$2,122	Inclusive of 2-day stay
Abdominoplasty	$1,857	$2,653	Inclusive of 3-day stay
Rhinoplasty	$530	$1,326	Exclusive of overnight stay

Source: Association of Private Hospitals of Malaysia

www.hospitals-Malaysia.org

days. For updated information, see the **Ministry of Foreign Affairs** Web site at **www.kln.gov.my**; the ministry of tourism maintains an extensive site at **www.tourism.gov.my**.

OTHER PLACES

There is practically no country in the Far East that does not see some sort of future for itself as a medical or health tourism destination, whether regional or worldwide. Look around; read the business news from Asia. You will find that even **Bangladesh**, a nation long perceived in the West as locked in poverty, aspires to provide health care for foreigners. **The Philippines** is a destination for some. The clerk at my local post office, who is inquisitive, managed to learn enough about medical tourism from me in the course of a few transactions that she did some research and is heading to that country for dental work.

Calixto V. Chikiamco, a columnist for *The Manila Times*, wrote in February 2004 that "some scattered, private-sector efforts are being done to court foreign patients," notably by big name hospitals like **St. Luke's Medical Center in Manila, Asian Hospital in Alabang**, and **Makati Medical Center**. The leading eye clinic in the country, the **Asian Eye Center in Rockwell**, established by the world-renowned Felipe Tolentino, M.D., has its fair share of foreign patients. "However, these efforts are nowhere near what Thailand has done," wrote Chikiamco. He said lack of government support and "institutional obstacles have made medical tourism "another missed opportunity" for the Philippines. In an effort to catch up, the country launched a major effort to promote medical tourism in early 2006.

Foremost among other countries in the Far East that have status as a destination country for medical tourism is the island state of **Singapore**, just to the south of Malaysia and, briefly, part of the Malaysian Federation in the 1960s before declaring independence. Singapore hospitals draw as many patients from abroad as does Malaysia, and the city-state has been a regional hub for medical services longer than has Malaysia, due to its level of economic development.

Singapore is not what is meant when social scientists talk about "developing countries." It is relatively affluent, with per capita income closer to that of Japan or of a number of Western European countries than to that of its immediate neighbors. Singapore has had modern hospitals and infrastructure much longer than has Malaysia.

It is that very affluence that works against Singapore now, however, as it competes for international patients. Prices for medical services and surgery are generally higher in Singapore than in Thailand, Malaysia, or India. They are still substantially lower than in the United States or Western Europe, making Singapore worth considering for those people who have compelling reasons for going there other than price. Singapore medical facilities, doctors, and surgeons are certainly among the best in the world. **The Johns Hopkins—Singapore International Medical Centre (www.imc.jhmi.edu)**, founded by Johns Hopkins University in Baltimore, Maryland, provides advanced oncology/cancer treatment at a level that one would expect simply from its origin. Nearly 80 percent of its patients come from abroad, mostly from Malaysia, Indonesia, India, Sri Lanka, Pakistan, and the United Arab Emirates.

The government of Singapore maintains an outstanding Web portal, **Singapore Medicine (www.singaporemedicine.com)**, that is the best place to start for any patient from abroad interested in investigating the country's health-care facilities.

CHAPTER 11

Pick a Country...
Any Country

I n the absence of health insurance, any expensive medical care I might ever need or want will certainly cause me to look abroad, as I did for dental care. And though I would go again to Costa Rica in a heartbeat and would be comfortable with any of the country choices detailed thus far, I also will always look again at South Africa, and think, *maybe this time.*

This is no more than me telling you that if your circumstances are such that you will seek medical care far from home, it is okay to think about the possibility of going someplace you have always wished to visit. There are good doctors and bad doctors everywhere, as many patients and physicians have already noted in this book. Bearing in mind that your first need will be top medical care at a price you can afford and that your second need will be a safe and comfortable recuperation, it is reasonable and natural to also ask yourself, *and where would I like to go?*

For me, a trip to South Africa would be a return, one I have contemplated off and on since 1994 when Nelson Mandela was elected president of the country, bringing about at least the political end of racial separation, apartheid. I had lived in South Africa in 1976 for a year when I was 20. That year I learned more about life and love and people than in any other three years of my life I could pick at random. It is a country I did not think would survive the 20th century intact, but it did, and I would know it again if I could. And South Africa, against all odds, is emphatically on the medical tourism map, with fine dentists, doctors, surgeons, and first-class private medical facilities. I could have gone there for my full-mouth reconstruction, and I thought about it. But cost, not sentiment, was the paramount consideration and Costa Rica won out.

Each medical tourist has his or her own sentiment in travel, or personal wanderlust. Mine draws me to South Africa. Yours may draw you to any of the major medical tourism destinations I have already mentioned, or it may draw you elsewhere. Though the most popular medical tourism destinations for U.S. citizens thus far are in Central and South America and the Far East, those are not the only places to go. They are just the paths most traveled.

> Medical tourism started to take off in about 2001, benefiting from international media attention.

SOUTH AFRICA

For all the extraordinary changes that have swept across **South Africa** since I was there, of most importance to any prospective medical tourist are some things that have not changed. Long gone are the days when the white minority population enjoyed arguably the highest economic standard of living in the world, but the country is still the richest in Africa, producing nearly a quarter of the continent's goods and services. The cities are modern, as are the private medical facilities.

Tourism, which languished in the 1990s, is on the rise. Overseas visitors number more than two million yearly, triple that of a decade ago when the country emerged from apartheid and international sanctions were lifted. Medical tourism, principally for cosmetic surgery and dentistry, started to take off in about 2001, benefiting from international media exposure. There was something irresistible first to British journalists, then to Americans, about reporting the success of medical tourism in Africa. An incongruously named medical tourism startup, **Surgeon and Safari (www.surgeon-and-safari.co.za)**, was the first big success story; "Seek out beauty, take in the beasts," was the perhaps inevitable headline in the *Financial Times* of London. "Silicone Safaris" was featured on the cover of the *Financial Mail*. At CNN, the story was billed as "Beauty and the Bush." Surgeon and Safari has also been profiled in *The Seattle Times*, *The Washington Post*, *The Wall Street Journal*, *Forbes*, and *Newsday*, among others.

The lure, besides excellent surgeons and medical care, is Africa itself. Most cosmetic surgery patients extend their stays for the scenery, or actual safaris. There are a number of medical tourism companies in the country, founded in the wake of the success of Surgeon and Safari.

Shopping around, as always, makes sense. Though most people who visit South Africa for cosmetic surgery work through medical tourist companies, it is possible to plan your own trip. South African surgeons do have their own Web sites. **The Association of Plastic and Reconstructive Surgeons of Southern Africa (APRSSA; www.plasticsurgeons.co.za)** has a comprehensive Web site with a directory of board-certified surgeons and advice for patients from overseas.

Overall, South Africa is not the cheapest medical tourism destination in the world. **Prices for surgery and procedures are higher than in Asia or Central and South America, averaging perhaps 50 percent of those in the United States. The trip is long—24 to 28 hours of travel time from the United States.** Airfare from the United States is expensive; figure $1,500 for rough planning purposes.

South Africa makes more sense for Europeans than it does for most Americans. But if your budget has room, you have the time, and Africa is in your dreams...by all means, South Africa is an option worth considering.

EASTERN EUROPE

The countries of **Eastern Europe** have gradually emerged as medical-tourism destinations over the last ten years. **Poland, Hungary,** and the **Czech Republic**, in particular, draw cosmetic surgery and dental patients from across Western Europe. The three were among those admitted to the European Union (EU) in 2004; the increased ease of travel and economic integration within an expanded EU seems certain to benefit medical tourism ventures in the less developed economies of the east. However, the phenomenon has been mostly regional and limited by the fact that Western European countries have near-universal health care.

There is some consternation in the United Kingdom about medical tourism and the effect it is having or may have on the National Health Service, but the ongoing discussion is more about the threat or promise of India than it is about Eastern Europe. In all of Europe, perhaps it is German cosmetic surgeons and dentists who express the most alarm about medical tourism, in much the same vein as some of their peers in

Texas might talk about U.S. residents going to Mexico. Germany is an easy drive to clinics and medical centers in Poland and Hungary.

But Eastern Europe remains comparatively undiscovered and unexplored by Americans. Overall, roughly 40 percent of all international tourists from the United States head for Europe, but only a tenth or so of them venture farther east than Austria or Berlin. Few of them thus far are medical tourists. Medical tourism in Eastern Europe is promoted primarily by individual private clinics and medical centers via the Internet and there is, as yet, no body of information available regarding patient experiences as there are for the Far East or Central and South America. The available evidence, however, indicates that there are medical tourism destinations in Eastern Europe that are competitive on both quality and price with those in the Far East and South America. Certainly Europeans are taking advantage of them, and U.S. medical tourists who are Europhiles may want to explore their options in the EU and eastward, all the way to **Moscow** and **St. Petersburg**.

For those who wish to go this route—at least from the United States—the path is not as well marked as it is to other places. If it is possible, I urge even more care and diligence in investigating individual destinations and doctors than I have for other places—not because I distrust the medical communities of the countries mentioned, but because relatively less information is available, even casually.

Poland

The Associated Press withdrew the veil over medical tourism in Eastern Europe in November 2004, reporting "a rising number of Germans and others from Western Europe are traveling to Poland and other new EU members such as Hungary and Slovakia to pay less for plastic surgery, fertility treatment, and dental work."

The story focused mainly on **Poland**, where many doctors and dentists have gone into private practice because of low salaries offered by government-run hospitals. **Prices for cosmetic surgery and dental work are 40 to 70 percent less than in Germany and the United States**. The AP interviewed patients who were happy with the quality of work done. European

Union health officials noted that no statistics were available on medical tourism in Poland but expressed the view that it was on the increase in border towns such as **Szczecin**, a port just 10 miles from Germany and reachable by ferry from Denmark.

Interested patients can easily find English-language Web sites for Poland cosmetic surgeons and dentists. One example is **Artplastica (www.artplastica.pl)**, advertising itself as "one of the biggest and the most modern private centers specializing in plastic surgery in Poland." Recovery accommodations are available and described on surgeon and dentist Web sites. Packages and arrangements are also available through some medical tourism companies, primarily those based in the United Kingdom. For rough planning purposes, roundtrip airfare to the region ranges from $500 to $800 from major U.S. cities. Travel time is 8 to 12 hours.

Hungary

The success of Hungarian dentists in attracting patients from the West has been perhaps the most widely reported medical tourism story coming out of the region. The *International Herald Tribune* noted the phenomenon in May 2005 in a story that was mostly about Hungary but generalized about the rest of the region.

"There are no exact numbers, but it is a booming business in places like the former Eastern bloc countries—both for doctors and dentists, as well as for the tour operators in countries like Ireland, Britain, and Denmark who help organize the trips," the paper said. One patient from Ireland's trip to a Hungarian dentist was summarized as follows:

> He toured the ancient castle in Budapest. He had dental bridges and fillings put in. He stayed in a luxury apartment overlooking the Danube. He had daily inhalation treatments at an asthma cave. He played golf and ate goulash. "I've been all over and the total cost—including the airfare—will be far less than what dental would cost me at home," he said, in a tidy waiting room, just after his final dental appointment in downtown Budapest. "I would recommend this in a second."

Most patients come from Germany, Austria, and the United Kingdom, the *Tribune* said, with just "a handful" traveling from the United States. That number seemed certain to increase, however, after *USA Today* reported on the high quality and low cost of Hungarian dental work, even listing contact information for specific dental clinics.

One happy patient indicated he had paid $6,000 for dental work that would have cost him $43,000 in the United States. The *USA Today* story, headlined "The inciDENTAL tourist," prompted at least one angry letter from a U.S. dentist, criticizing the article for treating dental care as a commodity and questioning whether standards in other countries met those in the United States. But the damage, if one could call it damage, was done. Hungary was on the medical tourism radar, at least.

> Budapest has actually been a health tourism destination for centuries.

Hungarian medical centers also offer cosmetic surgery, corrective eye surgery, and other medical procedures at **prices competitive with those in Poland**. A growing number of facilities have English-language Web sites and promote services through Western medical tourism companies. **Budapest** is widely referred to as "The Paris of Eastern Europe," and has actually been a health tourism destination for centuries—its mineral springs and spas are world famous. If any country in Eastern Europe can emerge as an international center of medical tourism, as opposed to a regional destination, Hungary's chances seem well above average.

The Czech Republic

What is true for Hungary and Poland is also true for the **Czech Republic**—though Czech doctors apparently expected more of an increase in medical tourism after their country joined the EU than materialized, according to *The Prague Post* in a July 2005 story.

"Beyond niche markets like spas, dentistry and elective treatments, EU membership has not yet resulted in a flood of West Europeans eager to book Prague clinics—much to the chagrin of many Czech doctors who hoped their fortunes would be sealed," the paper reported. Perhaps expectations were unrealistic. Dentistry and elective surgery are precisely the niches that would be expected to gain the most, and they have. *The Post* reported that a dozen new cosmetic surgery clinics have opened in the past three years. Czech medical facilities, doctors, and dentists market on the Internet, and through medical tourism companies.

Any Country

And what is true for Hungary, Poland, and the Czech Republic is true for much of the rest of Eastern Europe, only perhaps less so, at least insofar as its appeal to the Western market for its medical services. The nations directly bordering the more economically developed countries of Western Europe have the significant advantage of proximity and recognition of the market, though they have yet to take full advantage. But other countries in the region hope to capitalize on medical tourism. **Greece**, **Cyprus**, **Lithuania**, **Latvia**, **Estonia**, **Bulgaria**, and **Turkey** have all recognized the possibilities and one can find clinics, medical centers, doctors, surgeons, and dentists in each country. Further east, **Russia** is a destination with a reputation for quality and some of the lowest advertised prices for elective medical procedures in the world.

If I appear to give Eastern Europe short shrift, it is only because prospective medical tourists who are researching destinations will find that there is less information casually available about medical services than there is on other countries in other regions, at least as of this writing. From the perspective of a prospective patient in the United States, one would like to see some more in the way of centralized comprehensive Internet resources in English, perhaps under the auspices of the medical associations in the various countries. It is perhaps ironic that they do not now exist in nations that were known not so long ago for the centralized planning of their entire economies.

CHAPTER 12

Future Shock?

M edical tourism is not going away. Will competition be ferocious? Will overseas prices stay comparatively low? Will services get even better?

All indicators say yes to all three. International hospital companies have invested hundreds of millions of dollars in building world-class medical facilities abroad, and are increasingly marketing their services in the United States and Europe. The options they offer are attractive to individual patients for elective medical procedures and, in time, will be attractive to insurers as well. That the United States' medical system can not compete on price internationally is inarguable. Without even going below the surface, the difference in costs between the United States and any of the countries mentioned in this book is too great to make up by any conceivable adjustment. Prices for comparable surgery and care abroad will remain a fraction of what they are and will be in the United States.

Just how big might medical tourism get, and at what point will the health-care systems in the United States or even in other developed nations begin to feel its impact? In the market for elective cosmetic surgery, as we've seen, there has already been an effect. While some U.S. surgeons still warn against the dangers of going overseas for cosmetic surgery, others acknowledge that a lot of potential patients can't afford U.S. prices. Some U.S. surgeons are beginning to partner with overseas surgeons and medical facilities or are opening branch offices in the Caribbean or Central and South America. The long-term solution, says Harpal Singh, M.D., chairman of Fortis Healthcare in India, lies in partnerships: "It'll be mutually beneficial for both them and us."[1]

PENT-UP DEMAND

The potential market for lower-cost cosmetic surgery and procedures is enormous and mostly untapped. A February 2004 poll commissioned by the American Society for Aesthetic Plastic Surgery indicated that nearly one-quarter of all Americans and one-third of all American women say they would consider having cosmetic procedures.[2] Nearly 58 percent of Americans expressed a favorable view of cosmetic surgery. A 2004 poll conducted jointly by *Parenting* magazine and America Online said that *if money were of no influence*, 77 percent of mothers would wish to undergo cosmetic surgery in order to restore pre-childbirth figures.[3]

U.S. surgeons recognize the market. In fact, one of the arguments they used in fighting a proposed tax on cosmetic procedures in Illinois in 2005 was that it amounted to a levy on middle-class, working women. But there is a gap between their prices for surgery and what a substantial number of potential patients are willing to pay. The bulk of the growth in the U.S. market for cosmetic procedures for several years has been in lower-cost, less-invasive stopgap procedures such as Botox injections and cosmetic fillers. The desire to serve more patients at the "low end" of the market certainly is a catalyst to innovation by U.S. surgeons and researchers, with various new procedures coming out all the time. But there are, as yet, no inexpensive substitutes for the basic surgical procedures—face-lifts, liposuction, tummy tucks, and the like.

> 77 percent of mothers said they would wish to undergo cosmetic surgery to restore their pre-childbirth figures.

It certainly seems possible, even likely, that there will come a time when medical tourism will have become a force for change in the national health-care systems of the West, and that time likely will be when large health insurers and governments of the United States and Europe begin embracing medical tourism and bringing it into their systems. Such efforts are already being made and, in terms of holding down or lowering costs, it makes sense that this will happen, eventually. In terms of politics, culture, and the impact such steps will have on entrenched and powerful interests in developed countries, the safest guess, probably, is that change will arouse strong feelings and probably some resistance from the medical community, as well as calls for reform.

Doctors and hospitals in the United States, in particular, could counter that any significant "off shoring" or outsourcing of care will weaken the existing system to the detriment of all. The Raleigh, North Carolina *News & Observer* quoted a trustee of the American Medical Association concerning a story about a man going overseas for surgery he could not afford at home. "The American Medical Association would find it most unfortunate that an American, or a North Carolinian...would need to go out of his country and community to get the health care he needs," Rebecca Patchin, M.D., told the newspaper. "This is a sign that our health-care system in this country is broken. We need to fix it."[4]

I do not know anyone who would argue with the thought, but no "fix" appears to be in sight. The "brokenness" of the U.S. health-care system is far beyond my scope; that medical tourism might be part of the solution as well as being a symptom of a problem is an open debate.

FOR THE U.S.—BILLIONS IN SAVINGS

In July 2005, the World Bank published a policy paper suggesting that a "simple" change in insurance benefits in the United States would create incentives for consumers to travel for health care."[5] For just 15 highly tradable, low-risk treatments, the annual savings to the United States would be $1.4 billion, even if only one in ten patients who need these treatments went abroad, the report says. "Half of these annual savings would accrue to the Medicare program alone."

The 15 low-risk procedures were defined using the following criteria:

• The surgery constitutes treatment for a non-acute or non-traumatic condition, meaning that it is not an emergency.
• The patient must be able to travel without significant pain or inconvenience.
• The surgery must be fairly simple and commonly performed with insignificant rates of post-operative complications.
• The surgery requires minimal on-site follow-up treatment.

- The surgery generates minimal laboratory and pathology reports.
- The surgery results in minimal immobility to the patient during recovery.

The 15 procedures identified as fitting these criteria and immediately appropriate for medical tourism are:

- Knee surgery
- Shoulder surgery
- Prostate surgery
- Tubal ligation
- Hernia repair
- Skin lesion excision
- Adult tonsillectomy
- Hysterectomy
- Hemorrhoid removal
- Rhinoplasty (plastic surgery on the nose)
- Bunionectomy
- Cataract extraction
- Varicose vein surgery
- Glaucoma procedures
- Eardrum surgery

All of these procedures can be done more cost-effectively abroad, even including travel costs, according to the report.

Unlike TRICARE, the U.S. health-care program for military retirees and their families, Medicare will not pay benefits outside of the United States. Most private medical insurance plans do not, either, other than for emergencies or for out-of-network services. But there is no financial incentive for a U.S. resident with Medicare or private health-care insurance to travel abroad for non-elective surgery or medical treatment, even if the surgery or treatment will cost the insurance company far less. For the consumer as it now stands, it creates out-of-pocket costs in either instance. The paper goes to some lengths in attempting to quantify everything that might go into making a health-care choice, but the argument boils down to this: The difference in price between the United States and some other countries for common medical procedures is so large that insurers would save a lot of money if they would pay for patients to go abroad for medical care, including covering travel costs and even offering incentives to offset the inconvenience and perceived additional risk. The paper's authors attempt to quantify the cost of inconvenience and risk, assigning dollar values to what they call the "psychological cost" of going overseas for care (perhaps much as an insurance company would), and sketching out specific examples of how such a system might work.

For example, they put forth the case of an American needing knee surgery that would cost $10,000 in the United States. In Hungary (the country is chosen arbitrarily, I presume) the cost of the surgery and travel was put at $1,500. The "psychological cost" is arbitrarily set at $1,000, bringing the total cost of going to Hungary for this hypothetical knee surgery to $2,500.

In the United States, the authors say, a consumer likely would pay $2,000 out-of-pocket of the $10,000 total cost, assuming a uniform 20 percent coinsurance rate and, for simplicity, a zero deductible. The insurance company would pay the balance of $8,000.

On the other hand, if the consumer chose to go to Hungary, under the authors' scenario he or she would be reimbursed 80 percent of the foreign price inclusive of travel and psychological costs ($2,500). So the patient would get $2,000 from the insurance company to cover actual medical and travel costs of $1,500, and would come out $500 ahead after surgery! The insurance company would make a net monetary gain of $6,000.

It would be naïve to think that U.S. insurance companies are not doing the same math; the potential savings is too great for them to ignore. Consumers also stand to benefit. The only big financial losers in the equation above, of course, are the doctors and hospitals that make up the U.S. medical system.

"This is a billion-dollar industry. Who ever thought that you would outsource the doctor? But that is what we are doing," Clyde Prestowicz, author of *Three Billion New Capitalists: The Great Shift of Wealth and Power to the East*, said in an August 2005 interview at the Institute of

International Studies at the University of California at Berkeley.[6]

It is perhaps just a matter of time before medical insurers start introducing medical tourism options to their health plans. In fact, I have heard that it is already being done in individual cases—that insurers can be persuaded by patients to pay the full cost of a trip abroad for medical care rather than pay much more in the United States. It is not a simple matter, as the World Bank authors suggest, for any of this to happen on a large scale. Insurers will have to become convinced that quality is as good abroad as it is in the United States. That is the main reason that international hospitals are seeking (and receiving) JCAHO accreditation, which holds them to the same standards as U.S. medical facilities. Accreditation is something that insurance companies (and government officials) understand. According to India's *Central Chronicle*, "It is believed the only reason that the National Health Scheme of the U.K. decided to not direct its patients to Indian hospitals was because of the lack of accreditation and standardization." The Apollo Hospitals Group in Delhi was the first Indian hospital to qualify. At least a dozen others applied in 2005.

Patients will have to be convinced, as well. But as the authors point out, not only is medical tourism on the rise, many U.S. patients are already accustomed to being treated by foreign-born and foreign-trained doctors even in the United States. More than a quarter of all doctors working in the United States are international medical graduates, according to the American Medical Association. And the top eight countries of origin for foreign-born doctors in the United States are developing countries—India, the Philippines, Cuba, Pakistan, Iran, Korea, Egypt, and China.

> U.S. patients are already accustomed to being treated by foreign-born and foreign-trained doctors.

There are also, of course, a host of legal and bureaucratic issues involved, plus the likelihood that the stakeholders in the U.S. medical-services system—hospitals, doctors, and employees prominent among them—are not going to like any of this one bit.

It would not take much to turn it all into a national debate, particularly when some people seize on the notion that outsourcing medical care—outsourcing the American doctor—might, in the long run, help save Medicare and help the United States keep down the cost of taking care of an aging population. In the September 2005 issue of *The Futurist*, a magazine dedicated to serving as a neutral clearinghouse of ideas, Prof. Konrad Kressley of the University of South Alabama's International Studies Department speculated that, in time, the United States will partly outsource long-term care.[7] "While the idea of sending American nursing-home residents overseas appears outlandish, the imperatives as well as preconditions are well in place," he wrote, pointing out that United States retirement communities are already flourishing in Mexico, Costa Rica, and South American countries—and even on cruise ships. Lower costs have made retirement abroad an attractive option for many older Americans who no longer find Florida or the U.S. Southwest affordable."It is a short hop from seagoing care to land-based care in Asia for elderly and disabled Americans and Europeans. The current successful out-sourcing for acute care is easily translatable into long-term chronic care. Chronic care is labor intensive, so outsourcing to lower-labor-cost coun-tries would generate savings for customers while providing meaningful employment for the host population."

Many people will find shipping America's elderly and infirm off to Asia for long-term care "inappropriate," Kressley acknowledges. But that does not mean it will not happen, to the extent that some patients and their families will make that choice.

If faced with the decision myself, and I am only 49, would I choose a frugal Sun Belt retirement over a more expansive one in Costa Rica, or Brazil, or Thailand? I can not say. What seems certain is that I, and everyone else, will have options that as yet can only be barely imagined. The farther out one projects the future of medical tourism, the likelier it is of being far wrong, and to the point of silliness.

The unknowns are enormous. As opposed to quoting people who look 10 or 20 years into the future and see borderless free trade for medical services, with the bulk of non-emergency care migrating to the Far East,

I could cite those who foresee, not at all impossibly, that globalization will grind to a halt, even reverse, due to scarcity of resources for development. Much of what is medical tourism, as an example, is dependent on the continued availability of relatively inexpensive international air travel. I would not care to speculate about the price of jet fuel in 2020. We could all be marooned in our hometowns, from Houston to Hyderabad; or we could be flitting about the planet with rented atomic-powered personal jetpacks. Who is to say?

But it is reasonable to look out over the next couple of years, anyway, without getting too crazy about it, and make some short-range predictions.

1. Medical tourism will grow at a healthy rate, perhaps 15-20 percent year over year. In the United States consumer awareness will outpace growth—more potential consumers will become aware of the phenomenon as marketing from abroad and by medical tourism companies increases over the next decade.

2. To the dismay of doctors' organizations, insurers in the United States will experiment with offering overseas care options for some procedures, and incentives for choosing less expensive overseas options. Some hospitals with international accreditation will gain "in-network" status with insurers.

3. Investment from the United States in hospitals and care abroad will accelerate.

4. The long-running debate over health care in the United States will come to the forefront again during the presidential campaign of 2008. Candidates will cite medical tourism as a phenomenon that demonstrates how the U.S. health-care system is flawed and broken. However, there will be no consensus on how to lower costs, make health care more available in the United States, and no viable candidate will suggest that medical tourism is in any way a solution to the problem. No candidate will suggest opening Medicare to allow pay-

ments to doctors and facilities outside the United States; or, if one does, a political firestorm will erupt.

5. In the United Kingdom, the National Health Service (NHS) will cautiously accept some Indian hospitals for outsourcing surgery and procedures, as the hospitals gain international accreditation.

6. In the Far East, Thailand will continue to benefit the most by growth in medical tourism, thanks to its head start and widespread recognition. India's prospects will receive a boost from the agreements with the NHS. India's success is more tied to the extent to which it can reach agreements with international and U.S. insurers, to increased marketing, and to the development of a tourism infrastructure.

7. Medical tourism in South and Central American countries will boom despite the comparative lack of government support because of their natural advantage, proximity to the United States market. In particular, south-of-the-border cosmetic surgery will continue to grow. Growth is dependent on continued improvements in infrastructure and private and foreign investment, however.

8. Someone will get the bright idea of operating medical tourist cruise ships in international waters offshore from the United States, principally for cosmetic surgery. I'm surprised this hasn't happened already.

9. Eastern Europe medical tourism will remain off the beaten path for U.S. residents but will continue to grow for those living in the European Union.

10. Cooperation between hospitals and doctors in the United States and their counterparts overseas will grow, prompted by insurers, medical tourism companies, and the needs of medical tourism patients for after-care.

This is a rather modest set of predictions, and all bets are off in the event of, for example, a regional or global pandemic, substantial increases in incidents of terrorism, or international economic crisis. Nonetheless, I would expect them to mostly hold up through the end of the decade, barring substantial reform or change in the U.S. health-care system, which history suggests is unlikely. Overwhelmingly, the tendency is toward incremental change. There are no small changes, however, that can make the U.S. medical system competitive on price. Even if all Americans had health insurance, those who want cosmetic surgery or elective procedures would continue to go overseas, and insurers would still have a compelling financial interest in developing overseas care as an option for patients. By a number of estimates from different countries, medical tourism is growing by about 15 percent a year. There is nothing on the immediate horizon to suggest that it will not steadily grow.

***

In the spring of 2004, I went to Costa Rica and came back with a new smile, a mouthful of perfect white teeth that, hypothetically, would have cost between $18,000 and $30,000 in the United States. My total bill for dental work in Costa Rica came to $8,290. Meals, lodging, and a little sightseeing cost me about $800; airfare would have been about $400, but I paid with frequent flier miles. It was my last, best option, I thought. I know now that perhaps I could have gotten the work done even cheaper, but I do not quarrel with the success of my results.

But even I still shake my head a little at the thought of what I did. It is clearly not for everyone. In a changing world, however, it is an option for many—often a last, best option.

1 The Times of India, New Delhi, India. Medical tourism: India's new tool to cause heart-burn in U.S. Dec. 25, 2005.

2 American Society for Aesthetic and Plastic Surgery. ASAPS Cosmetic Surgery Attitude Study. Feb. 14, 2004. Available at www.surgery.org.

3 Parenting Magazine. Oct. 2004.

4 The News & Observer, Raleigh, N.C. Americans increasingly find health care abroad. Vicki Cheng. Sept. 23, 2004.

5 World Bank Policy Research Working Paper 3667: Does health insurance impede trade in health care services? Aaditya Mattoo and Randeep Rathindran. July 2005.

6 Clyde Prestowitz Interview: Conversations with History; Institute of International Studies, UC Berkeley. Aug. 2005.

7 The Futurist. Aging and public institutions. Konrad M. Kressley. Sept.-Oct. 2005.

Afterword

A Bangladeshi, a Brit, an Arab, and a New Yorker were sitting in a doctor's waiting room...

What could be a preamble for an off-color joke is in reality the tangible face of the medical tourism phenomenon. What brings together such a rich mélange of people to a medical facility thousands of miles from the comfort of their homes? In fact, their motivation is as diverse as their cultures, languages, and geography.

The Bangladeshi seeks an alternative to the less-developed medical system in his own country. He comes for *quality*.

The British woman undergoing radiation therapy for her breast cancer is side-stepping the long queue in England's socialized health-care scheme. She comes for *access*.

The affluent Emirati from the United Arab Emirates is seeing four doctors in one morning with a personal interpreter/valet in tow and a steaming cup of Starbucks coffee in his hand. He comes for *service*.

Then there is the New Yorker. What on earth is he doing here? What has possessed this 55-year-old upper-middle-class stockbroker from one of the most cosmopolitan cities in the world to leave behind arguably the most sophisticated medical system on the planet to have surgery in Asia? He is one of 42 million uninsured Americans who is self-employed, not rich, not poor, old enough to need his prostate removed, but not old enough to qualify for Medicare. And he does not want to pay the high price for private medical insurance. He comes for *price*.

But the Americans can not be sold on price alone. Our friend from New York is a case in point. Of course, the price was 80 percent less than that of the U.S. quotes he got. But being a day-trader, he knows his research. He knows what he wants—a cutting-edge minimally invasive laser procedure for prostate removal by a surgeon who has done the procedure more often than anyone else in the world, in a hospital that is of international standard that could take him right away. His search brought him to Asia. He came for *quality*...and *access*...and *service*...and *price*.

As an American who has lived in Asia for over a decade, I can safely say that we Americans are a demanding bunch. And it is truly a leap of faith to trust your health to a doctor that you have never met at a hospital you have never seen in a country you have to first find on a map.

This is the value then of Jeff Schult's excellent guide to the world of medical tourism. Jeff has scoured the hot-spots of medical tourism, talked to the patients, Googled the Internet to within an inch of its life, and taken the plunge himself into overseas health care. The result is a balanced, unbiased, and thoughtful guide for the informed consumer. *Beauty from Afar* is an entertaining and practical handbook that includes important considerations that any prospective medical tourist would...and should...consider before making the "leap."

I thought I knew a lot about the subject, having lived it for 10 years. Jeff has opened a whole new world of possibilities, and he has made me a student again. I am convinced more than ever that medical tourism is not a fad. It is not about "cheap" health care. It is about smart, well-informed people looking for quality service at a reasonable price in a world where distances and lines drawn on a map are not the barriers they once were.

Decisions about your health are important. As this book has instructed, do your own research; make smart, informed decisions. Maybe you can narrow the leap of faith to more of a hop.

Healthy Travels!

Curtis J. Schroeder
Group Chief Executive Officer
Bumrungrad International
Bangkok, Thailand

INDEX

I

India, 20, 24, 59, 165-66, 168,171-79, 185, 189
    future and, 195, 200, 202-3
    and history of medical tourism, 63, 70-72
    infrastructure of, 172-73, 175
    marketing medical tourism in, 166,
        172-73, 175-76
    media on, 165, 172-73, 177, 179
    non-cosmetic procedures in, 26-27, 38,
        40, 85-87
    popularity of medical tourism in,
        36, 38-40
    tourism in, 172, 175
    travel and, 110, 112
    U.S. affiliates in, 173-74
injectible fillers, 32, 76, 196
International Society of Aesthetic
    Plastic Surgery, The (ISAPS), 55, 94, 131
Internet, 16-18, 24, 189-93, 208
    Brazil and, 92-93, 101, 103, 123, 126-27,
        129-33
    and cautions on medical tourism, 49-50
    cosmetic procedures and, 79, 84-85
    cosmetic surgery sites on, 92-95
    Costa Rica and, 99, 101, 104, 135-37,
        140-42, 150-52, 155, 162
    and definitions of medical tourism, 38-40
    dental care and, 16-17, 29
    Dominican Republic and, 44-46
    Eastern Europe and, 190-92
    Far East and, 166-68, 170, 173, 176, 178,
        180-82, 184-85
    general sites on, 91-92
    and history of medical tourism, 69-70
    and learning from overseas surgeons,
        56-57
    Mexico and, 100-101, 155-59, 162-63
    patient support sites on, 95-96
    and popularity of cosmetic surgery,
        32-33
    research and, 20, 29, 89-107, 167, 170
    search engines on, 91, 97-105
    travel and, 96-97, 114-15

J

Johns Hopkins-Singapore International
    Medical Centre, The, 185
Joint Commission on Accreditation of
    Healthcare Organizations (JCAHO),
    143-44, 167, 200
Jurassic Park (Crichton), 17-18

K

Kressley, Konrad, 201

L

Las Cumbres Inn Surgical Retreat 135-37,
    140-41, 150
Lev, Alejandro, 25, 142-43
liposuction/lipoplasty, 18-19, 25, 51, 81-83,
    99, 135, 196
    cost of, 16, 77-78, 183
    in Far East, 168, 183
    and popularity of medical tourism,
        32-35, 40
lower body lifts (belt lipectomies), 82

M

Macaya, Federico, 135, 137, 139
Makati Medical Center, 184
Making the Body Beautiful (Gilman), 71
Malaysia, 18, 20, 35, 54, 70, 85, 128, 166,
    169, 177-85
    geography of, 179-80
    infrastructure of, 178, 180, 185
    marketing medical tourism in, 177-78,
        180-82
    media on, 177-79
    rates for major procedures in, 182-83
    tourism in, 180-84
    travel and, 110, 112
malpractice insurance, 60
Martin, Ruben and Lorena, 139
Martino Resort & Spa, 138
meals, 59, 119, 174
    in Costa Rica, 138, 140-42, 204
medical tourism:
    cautions on, 43, 45, 49-57, 171
    coining of the term, 18-19
    controversy and confusion about, 47-48
    definitions of, 15, 38-40, 64
    family doctor consultations for, 52-53
    in future, 28, 194-205
    history of, 62-73, 138-39, 147-48, 150
    marketing of, 25, 34-35, 51, 54-55, 67,
        69-70, 126-29, 141-45, 150-51, 162,
        165-66, 168-70, 172-73, 175-78,
        180-82, 190-93, 202-3
    media on, 16, 18-20, 33-34, 70-72, 89,
        177-79, 184, 188, 197, 200
    popularity of, 25-27, 32-40, 46, 49, 149,
        158-59, 162, 166, 168, 170, 172-73,
        177-78, 184, 191-93, 200, 202-4
    research on, 20-21, 29, 50, 89, 96, 98,
        102-4, 151, 184